A Cultural History of Pregnancy

A Cultural History of Pregnancy

Pregnancy, Medicine and Culture, 1750–2000

Clare Hanson
Department of English
Loughborough University

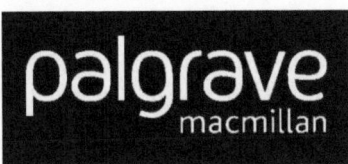

First published 2004 by
PALGRAVE MACMILLAN
Houndmills, Basingstoke, Hampshire RG21 6XS and
175 Fifth Avenue, New York, N. Y. 10010
Companies and representatives throughout the world

PALGRAVE MACMILLAN is the global academic imprint of the Palgrave Macmillan division of St. Martin's Press, LLC and of Palgrave Macmillan Ltd. Macmillan® is a registered trademark in the United States, United Kingdom and other countries. Palgrave is a registered trademark in the European Union and other countries.

ISBN 978-0-333-98644-8

This book is printed on paper suitable for recycling and made from fully managed and sustained forest sources.

A catalogue record for this book is available from the British Library.

Library of Congress Cataloging-in-Publication Data
Hanson, Clare.
    A Cultural History of Pregnancy: Pregnancy, Medicine, and Culture,
    1750–2000 / Clare Hanson.
        p. cm.
    Includes bibliographical references and index.
    ISBN 978-0-333-98644-8 (cloth)
        1. Pregnancy–Social aspects–Great Britain–History. 2. Pregnancy–Great Britain–Psychological aspects–History. 3. Obstetrics–Great Britain–History.
    I. Title.

RG556.H36 2004
618.2–dc22   2003070739

10   9   8   7   6   5   4   3   2
13 12 11 10 09 08 07 06 05

Transferred to Digital Printing 2005

Contents

List of Illustrations

Acknowledgements

Many colleagues have assisted me in the writing of this book. I am particularly grateful to Nicola Bradbury, Maroula Joannou and Imelda Whelehan, who generously read draft material and offered helpful criticism and advice. Mark Hanson read the complete typescript and provided much constructive criticism. Sarah Gamble gave early encouragement and put me on the track of the Haldanes. I am grateful to the staff of the Wellcome Library for the History and Understanding of Science for their friendly assistance, and in particular to Miriam Gutierrez-Perez for her help with visual material. The staff of the British Library have also been unfailingly courteous and helpful. My final thanks go to Antonia and Jack Hanson for their cheerful support.

A section of Chapter 4 first appeared in *Literature and History* 12, 2, Autumn 2003. I am grateful to the editors for permission to reproduce this material. I am also grateful to the Wellcome Medical Photographic Library for permission to reproduce the following images:

William Hunter, Plate XX, *The Anatomy of the Human Gravid Uterus* (artist unknown), 'A male-midwife suggestively examines a pregnant woman'
Thomas Rowlandson, 'Joanna Southcott the prophetess'
Lars Nilsson, '20-week foetus sucking thumb'
'Ultrasound scanning equipment'
Chris Nurse, 'Pregnancy'

A Note on Spelling

Throughout the text I have used the English spelling 'foetus', as this is the spelling used in the majority of the obstetric texts analysed here and it remains the preferred spelling in current British English. I have used the American spelling 'fetus', however, when quoting from modern scientific sources (for which it is the accepted spelling) or from American texts.

Introduction

In October 1791, Judith Milbanke wrote to her aunt, Mary Noel, reporting her suspicion that she was pregnant, after fifteen childless years of marriage and two miscarriages. Her situation was unusual in many respects. She was married to Ralph Milbanke, a Whig MP with whom she lived happily and who apparently put no pressure on her to bear children in order to continue the family line. She was actively involved in his political career, led a busy social life and, above all, was wealthy.[1] Yet, despite her privileged position, her pregnancy plunged her into the doubts and uncertainties which were then the inevitable concomitants of the condition. Her aunt's letters to her offer a vivid glimpse of the anxiety and indeterminacy which characterised the experience at a time when it was impossible to have a certain diagnosis until a child could literally be seen in the course of labour. In response to Judith's first letter, her aunt writes of her own agitation, speculates as to symptoms and enjoins the strictest secrecy for fear of ridicule if Judith's hopes should prove false. Her next letter reports consultations with friends about 'breeding women' who, like Judith, have a 'hungry feel, & then they are not sick'. By 9 November she writes, 'I now begin to think you certainly must be breeding, for you have every Symptom except sickness, & that is no proof as it often is occasion'd by a Stoppage.'[2] In the same letter she suggests that Judith should contact the fashionable *accoucheur* Dr Denman, giving her symptoms and asking his opinion as to whether or not she is pregnant. Two weeks later the rumour about Judith's pregnancy was out, but its status still remained uncertain. Even though quickening (the mother's first experience of foetal movements) was generally considered the most reliable sign of pregnancy, it could offer no certainty. So, on 2 December, Mary Noel remained fearful, writing, 'I found your very agreeable Kick-Shaw

1

of a letter here on my arrival last night which was a greater feast to me than my dinner... – but I wish you could have been more certain' (p. 401). It was not until mid-December, when Judith was four months pregnant, that she allowed her aunt to begin to think about the confinement. At this point Mary Noel again urged the use of an *accoucheur* such as Denman who attended 'the eminent', and even went as far as to have a consultation with him on Judith's behalf. Denman was reassuring: in particular, he 'did not know there was any necessity for your having more pains or worse time on account of your Age' (p. 411). Judith eventually gave birth to a daughter, Annabella, on 17 May 1792, attended by her aunt at Elemore Hall in the north of England. Annabella married Lord Byron in 1815, which is why we have a record of this pregnancy.[3]

Two hundred years later, the novelist Rachel Cusk described her first pregnancy in her memoir *A Life's Work: On Becoming a Mother*. Her account begins with a visit to the GP to tell him that she is pregnant: the reader infers that she knows this from a pregnancy testing kit, readily available from any chemist. Cusk then goes on a walking holiday in the Pyrenees and accidentally slips down a glacier. As she makes her way painstakingly to safety, she notices a gap which has begun to open up within her between fact and feeling: climbing back carefully despite her fear, she notes, 'what I feel, it seems, is no obstacle to what I am able to do'.[4] The next landmark is the ultrasound scan:

> Just wiggle your hips up and down, commands the sonographer, and we'll see if we can get it to move. On the computer screen beside the bed, a small, monochrome crustacean lies in a snowstorm of static ... Come on, the sonographer urges the creature harshly, let's see you move! She presses the scanner down harder on my stomach. The creature waves its thin arms as if distressed. (p. 24)

Cusk realises that the spectacle of the foetus moving is being produced not simply for medical reasons but also for 'my own entertainment', and she is given a photograph to take away, a trophy/totem image of the encounter. She is also given a copy of *Emma's Diary*, a fictional account of pregnancy produced by the National Health Service which is full of suggestions for the proper conduct of pregnancy, as are a plethora of other books and leaflets about pregnancy, which advise on diet, exercise, sleeping positions and making love. Cusk begins to resent the literature, with its 'ghoulish hints at the consequences of thoughtless actions. Eat pâté and your baby will get liver damage. Eat blue cheese and your baby will get listeria' (p. 29). As the pregnancy progresses, she feels 'despair' at her predicament, 'marooned as far from myself as I will ever be'. But it is not abstinence, nor the 'extremity' of her physical transformation, nor the strange pains she experiences which affect her most, but the loss of her privacy, which she describes in these terms:

> It is the population of my privacy, as if the door to my room were wide open and strangers were in there, rifling about, that I find hard to endure … I read newspaper reports of women in America being prosecuted for harming their unborn foetuses and wonder how this can be; how the body can become a public space, like a telephone box, that can unlawfully vandalise itself … it is as if some spy is embedded within me, before whose scrutiny I am guilty and self-conscious. It is not, I feel sure, the baby who exerts this watchful pressure: it is the baby's meaning for other people, the world's sense of ownership stating its claim. (pp. 34–5)

Despite the careful monitoring of this pregnancy, Cusk starts to bleed at eight months and is found to be suffering from undiagnosed placenta praevia (a potentially life-threatening condition, caused when the placenta covers all or part of the cervix). Her daughter is delivered by emergency caesarean section: Cusk 'recognises her immediately' from the scan of a few days earlier.

These two narratives, divergent in so many ways, offer a vivid illustration of the ways in which pregnancy is differently framed and experienced in different cultural contexts. Indeed, this is the premise with which this book begins: that the pregnant body (itself arguably a form of double embodiment) is doubly mutable. It is mutable in the obvious sense that it undergoes continuous physiological (and sometimes pathological) change, and mutable culturally, in that it is viewed through constantly shifting interpretive frameworks. These interpretive frameworks are constructed through the interrelation of medicine and culture, an interrelation which is complex and cannot be assimilated to a single theoretical model. For example, some developments in medical knowledge have their origin in the pursuit of a particular and well-defined scientific goal, which then has (unintended) effects on other areas of medical practice. Thus, in connection with pregnancy, when René Laënnec invented the stethoscope in 1819, it was used by his pupil Jacques Alexandre de Kergaradec to listen for the 'splashing' of the foetus in the amniotic fluid. Instead, he discovered the foetal heartbeat and thus provided what is still one of the most important monitoring tools for pregnancy. Auscultation (listening for the foetal heart) then became 'translated' into an acceptable component of obstetric practice, although within the strict constraints of modesty which framed the interaction between male doctor and pregnant patient in the nineteenth century. In other words, it became mediated by culture. On the other hand, some 'developments' in medicine have their primary origin not in medical enquiry, but in cultural pressures producing behaviour which is then assimilated into categories of 'disease' and 'treatment' by the medical profession: the so-called 'insanity of pregnancy', diagnosis of which flourished in the nineteenth century, is a good example of this process. For while medicine and culture can be considered discrete fields of knowledge, their boundaries are permeable: there is an osmotic relation between them.

This book explores changes in the cultural 'framing' of pregnancy in Britain over the last 250 years through an analysis of a range of medical and cultural texts. It draws on a range of sources which include obstetric and midwifery books, advice books for women, medico-social texts, literary texts, popular fiction and visual images. In line with the osmotic metaphor, no single type of source is privileged over the others: it is not assumed, for example, that the discourse of medical science has ontological priority over other discourses. The aim of this book is not to chart 'cultural responses' to changes in medical understanding, but to explore the ways in which medical, scientific, social and imaginative discourses work together to create an interpretive horizon which frames the understanding and experience of pregnancy at any given time. Such a horizon will be patchy in its influence and will also be internally fractured and contradictory, as the discourses which construct it, each with its own cultural history and investments, interrogate each other. For if no texts are 'outside' ideology, none is saturated by it. This is as true of medical texts as it is of works of social commentary or of literary texts. Indeed, as Jill Matus has pointed out, medical discourse can sometimes appear 'more open, exploratory and less ideologically obedient than fictive imaginings'.[5] None the less, because of the truth-claims attaching to medical discourse, it remains necessary to stress the fact that the language of medical science, although it struggles for objectivity, cannot escape the fact that, as a language, it is not value-free. As Evelyn Fox Keller has put it in a recent study of the gene, 'Like the rest of us, scientists are language speaking actors. The words they use play a crucial (and, more often than not, indispensable) role in motivating them to act ... By their words, their very landscapes of possibility are shaped.'[6]

It is also important to emphasise that in exploring the 'landscapes of possibility' created by discourses of pregnancy, this study is a history of ideas and cultural representations, and not an attempt to access what could be called 'the historical Real'. As E. Ann Kaplan has argued, in such areas as the conduct of pregnancy and of child-rearing, subjective experience – complex, contradictory and often unrecorded – is extremely difficult to recover.[7] In *The Captured Womb*, Ann Oakley makes a similar point, asking, 'Were pregnant women anxious? Were they more anxious in 1781 than in 1881 or 1981? We have no way of telling.'[8] But if we cannot recover subjective experiences, we can trace the discourses that have framed and inflected pregnancy, and in so doing disclose a history of the ideas that have shaped and informed experience. We can also register and analyse changes in the conduct and management of pregnancy, changes driven as much by social as by medical imperatives. We can thus trace, for example, the rise of obstetrics and the relationships which were established between the wealthy woman and her *accoucheur*/physician. Such relationships were, among other things, a means by which the independence of the pregnant woman could be protected. In the twentieth century, we can chart changing patterns in the state provision of medical care for pregnant women, as well as changes in relation to employment and leisure.

As indicated above, the texts examined in this book are drawn from three main categories: the medical; the medico-social; and the literary (although material which falls outside these categories is also included). The medical texts which are considered are primarily obstetric and midwifery textbooks and 'advice' books for pregnant women. The medico-social texts which are discussed take rather different forms in the nineteenth and twentieth centuries. In the nineteenth century, when scientific investigation was developing a new understanding of the relationship between mind and body, such texts were typically (though not always) written by medical specialists reflecting on the social implications of their findings. In the twentieth century, such texts were more often produced by committees reporting to the government. The authors of such reports included not only members of the medical profession, but also social scientists and statisticians, as well as lay members. The literary texts which are analysed include a range of popular as well as 'high' cultural texts. Within each field, the texts selected for discussion are those which engage most fully with the key concepts framing the understanding of pregnancy in a particular period. Of course, this begs the question how one determines which *are* the key concepts. In this study I have concentrated on those ideas which have had the most resonance across the discursive fields outlined above, for example, maternal irritability/sensibility, the insanity of pregnancy, eugenic motherhood, and so on.

As Milbanke's and Cusk's stories suggest, as the mechanism by which society reproduces itself, pregnancy is by no means a private matter, but is peculiarly susceptible to social intervention and control. Thus, at the macro level, reproduction throughout the period covered by this study has been considered critical to the strength and survival of the nation-state. In 1945, for example, when the birth rate was falling below replacement levels and it was projected that by 2020 the population would fall to 28 million, a Royal Commission was set up to consider the implications of this in a post-war context. It concluded, significantly, that the situation was dangerous not just for Britain, but also for the Commonwealth. It was considered that the question was 'not merely one of military strength and security' for Britain, but that it 'becomes merged in more fundamental issues of the maintenance and extension of Western values, ideas and culture'.[9] Accordingly, the Report suggested ways in which the state could intervene to encourage reproduction, recommending, for example, tax-breaks for those who had children. On a smaller scale, reproduction within the legal structure of marriage has been considered desirable for social stability, providing, among other things, a secure conduit for the transmission of property. The underwriting of family structure through inheritance law has been crucial here. Of course, legal provisions change in accordance with changing social needs and practices. In the eighteenth century, the dominant class was the landed gentry, who could transmit wealth and status to the next generation only by leaving an intact estate; hence their preference for the laws of primogeniture and entail. In the early nineteenth century, however, with the rise of a middle class with assets in liquid capital, the principle of divided inheritance began to be favoured, with assets more commonly distributed among heirs, including wives and daughters.[10] However, despite such changes, reproduction always takes place within a juridical context.

This is equally true at the micro level, in cases where pregnancy might appear to be a matter for one individual only. For example, if a woman becomes pregnant but wishes for an abortion, under current legislation she has a right to seek it without reference to anyone's wishes other than her own, whether she is married or single. Legally, she can have an abortion if the risks of continuing the pregnancy, in relation to her physical and mental health, are judged to be greater than those of terminating it.[11] This presents us with the familiar paradox whereby the individual's 'right to choose' must be protected by law. The possibility of choice, in what many consider a most private matter, exists only because the state has intervened to make this possible.

The intense legal activity which has accompanied recent developments in reproductive technology has therefore only made more visible what has always been the case: reproduction, like production and consumption, is a public as well as a private matter. None the less, despite this thread of continuity, there has been a major shift in the way pregnancy has been understood during the period covered by this book, a shift that is related in part to demographic change. From the eighteenth century until the 1870s, the UK population grew rapidly, giving rise to fears of overpopulation, most notoriously expressed by Thomas Malthus.[12] However, in the late 1870s, the birth rate began to fall and, by the end of the Second World War, as noted above, the predominant fear was of *de*population. The reasons for the fall in the birth rate were twofold. The first was increased knowledge about and access to contraception. Many commentators have seized on the fact that it was in the critical decade of the 1870s that Annie Besant and Charles Bradlaugh were prosecuted for selling Dr Knowlton's *Fruits of Philosophy*, a book giving contraceptive advice. The trial generated enormous publicity, and over the next twenty years over a million tracts giving contraceptive information were sold.[13] The dissemination of contraceptive information in the late nineteenth century probably had more impact on the birth rate than Marie Stopes' work in the 1920s. However, the period between 1880 and 1920 coincided with the first wave of feminism, and it was women's desire for greater independence which was the second major factor leading to a rapid reduction in family size.

The effects of this demographic revolution were far-reaching in relation to the conduct and experience of pregnancy. Previously, it had been expected that a fertile woman would bear around eight children during her reproductive life; thus each individual pregnancy was not critical in relation to the survival of the family. Moreover, given the conditions of pregnancy and childbirth, and the relatively few options for medical intervention, women and men expected to lose one or more of their children through miscarriage, stillbirth or death in early infancy. As historians have argued, this does not mean that their grief over the loss of an individual child would not have been as great as it is today, but it would have been differently inflected, because it was experienced in different medical, social and religious contexts. It is partly for these reasons that the primary interest of obstetrics from the eighteenth century to the early twentieth century was in the care of the mother, not the child. In his 1752 *Treatise on the Theory and Practice of Midwifery*, William Smellie articulated the golden rule which prevailed for 150 years: 'The mother's life is always to be more regarded than the safety of the child.'[14] It is still the case that when there is a conflict between the interests of mother and child, the mother's safety comes first, but the difference lies in Smellie's and his contemporaries' generally pragmatic acceptance of foetal death. However, at the beginning of the twentieth century, at the very moment when social commentators were beginning to take note of the falling birth rate, J.W. Ballantyne published a paper in the *British Medical Journal* which introduced a radically new perspective to the field of antenatal care. In his 'A Plea for a Pro-Maternity Hospital', Ballantyne argued for the establishment of specialised units which would be devoted to 'prenatal diagnosis and treatment'.[15] Significantly, he distinguished between those cases in which the 'maternal factor' was of prime importance and those in which 'antenatal therapeutics' came under consideration (in other words, the treatment of the unborn child via the mother). Ballantyne's article, which was extremely influential, marked the beginning of a shift in obstetric medicine, away from the health of the mother and towards the health of the foetus. This was made possible by a number of interlocking factors, most importantly the reduction in maternal mortality brought about by the gradual elimination of puerperal fever.[16] However, the new concern for foetal welfare was also clearly linked with the declining birth rate and with the prevalence of smaller families. To put it bluntly, the law of supply and demand was in operation: the successful outcome of a pregnancy became more important as pregnancy itself became scarcer. As we shall see, this is still more the case in the contemporary context of declining fertility and increased use of assisted conception.

As Ballantyne was well aware, his interest in antenatal therapeutics brought into sharp focus issues with which we are still struggling. What is the precise nature of the relationship between mother and foetus? How should we interpret and characterise it? To what extent can they be considered 'one flesh', as J.W. Sykes contended?[17] And what are the respective rights of the mother and foetus? In the eighteenth and nineteenth centuries, the dominant paradigm for the relationship was one which Ballantyne himself termed 'harmonious symbiosis': in other words, pregnancy was viewed as a state in which 'the unborn child and parent live together ... with mutual benefit'.[18] Thus the man-midwife John Grigg, in his 1789 *Advice to the Female Sex in General, Particularly those in a State of Pregnancy and Lying-in*, wrote that pregnancy was not only beneficial for the child, but that if women dutifully followed 'the progress of nature', their powers of both body and mind would be invigorated by pregnancy. The midwife Martha Mears, in her *The Midwife's Candid Advice to the Fair Sex; or the Pupil of Nature*, similarly argued that the condition of pregnancy brought a woman 'nearer to the perfection of her being; and, instead of disease, affords a much stronger presumption of health and security'.[19] A competing model, which gained ground in the twentieth century, was that of parasitism, or a view of pregnancy as a 'nine months' malady' which was prejudicial to the mother, 'a condition of tension or strain' as Ballantyne put it. This view is expressed with admirable clarity by Margery Spring Rice in her study *Working-class Wives*, in which she suggests that 'it is well known that the unborn baby takes what it needs from its mother so far as such requirements can be found in her body; therefore it is the woman's reserves of nutriment and vitamins which suffer during the nine months of pregnancy, if her diet is inadequate'.[20] A third model which is emerging from current studies of foetal growth offers a more 'competitive' view of the relationship between mother and foetus. It suggests that where nutritional resources are scarce, it is by no means certain that the foetus will automatically take all that it needs from the mother. In such conditions, more complex mechanisms of exchange and adaptation may come into play, and the foetus may be forced to prioritise some aspects of its development at the expense of others.[21]

These different models have overlapped and coexisted throughout the period covered by this study. For example, Thomas Denman proposed a 'parasitic' model of pregnancy in his 1788 *Introduction to the Practice of Midwifery* (anticipating Margery Spring Rice by 150 years) while the much older model of 'harmonious symbiosis' continues to underpin contemporary booklets of advice to mothers published in association with the British Medical Association.[22] The same is true in relation to the question of maternal and foetal rights: we can trace broad shifts in perceptions and attitudes, but at any given moment differing perspectives will coexist. In relation to this issue, however, the overall pattern, as we might expect, has been one of increasing concern for the foetus. This has been particularly marked with the advent of routine ultrasound scanning and with recent developments in foetal medicine: together these have brought into being the 'foetal patient', who is often considered to have rights almost identical to those of the child *ex utero*.[23] Anti-abortionists have, of course, long campaigned for the 'right to life' from the moment of conception, and debate over the question of when life begins has intensified as reproductive technologies have made it possible to freeze and store embryos. Yet though we might assume that such a concern with the rights of the embryo/foetus is an almost exclusively twentieth-century phenomenon, this is far from the case. In the late eighteenth and early nineteenth centuries, obstetricians were much exercised by the ambiguous legal status of the unborn child. In his 1837 work *An Exposition of the Signs and Symptoms of Pregnancy*, W.F. Montgomery wrote at some length on the contradictory situation whereby an embryo had a legal existence from the moment of its conception in relation to inheritance law, whereas in cases where a pregnant woman was 'pleading her belly' in an effort to escape capital punishment, the child was deemed to have such an existence only from the moment of quickening.[24]

In addition to the models described above of the relationship between mother and unborn child (symbiosis, parasitism and competition), a further trope which has long dominated discussions and representations of pregnancy is that of 'nature'. The nature–culture opposition has been played out on a number of levels, which have both political and experiential implications. The issue is political in that pregnancy poses a particular challenge to the medicalisation of the body which has characterised post-Enlightenment Western society.[25] Is pregnancy a natural or a pathological state? The answer is not as straightforward as it may seem. We can divide pregnancy into the categories of normal and abnormal (as Ballantyne does), normal pregnancy being considered non-pathological. The difficulty is that, in any given pregnancy, the normal can tip over into the abnormal very quickly, which means that there is a strong *prima facie* case for the medical monitoring of all pregnancies. On the other hand, many women find such monitoring intrusive and demeaning, with the result that it has a negative impact on their experience of pregnancy and even, it has been argued, on its outcome. In general, the issue has tended to split the medical profession along gendered lines, with midwives defending the line of least intervention (nature) and man-midwives/obstetricians advocating intervention (culture). (This is not always the case, a notable exception being the male obstetrician Grantly Dick Read's promotion of 'natural childbirth' in the 1930s.)

Paradoxically, both sides in this debate have consistently attempted to align their practices with 'nature'. In the later eighteenth century, for example, when there was a particularly fierce antagonism between midwives and man-midwives, male practitioners such as Grigg and Alexander Hamilton went out of their way to advocate 'an exact, patient attendance of the efforts of Nature' in pregnancy and child-birth, with the result that their rhetoric, if not their clinical practice, became almost indistinguishable from that of contemporary midwives such as Martha Mears and Elizabeth Nihell.[26] A professed respect for nature (or Nature) was a guarantee of respectability, even delicacy – crucial attributes, of course, for a male practitioner who wished to make his mark in obstetric medicine. Pushing the point further, at certain critical moments in medical history the rhetorical opposition between nature and culture can be seen to dissolve and collapse entirely. A good example is in the debate over James Simpson's use of chloroform for a patient in labour in 1847. This caused a furore, with many accusing him of impiety and of posing a challenge to the biblical commandment, 'in sorrow thou shalt bring forth children' (Genesis 3:16). Simpson responded eloquently and energetically to his critics, pointing out that 'If God has *beneficently* vouchsafed to us a means of mitigating the agonies of childbirth, it is His evident intention that we should employ these means.' Further, in answer to his main opponent, Professor Meigs of Philadelphia, he wrote:

> The truth is, all the tendencies of man, in a civilised state of society, are to intermeddle with and change, and, as he conceives, improve the action of almost every function in the body. And each such improvement has, at the time of its introduction, been, like the practice of anaesthesia, very duly denounced as improper, impious, &c., &c.[27]

Simpson's remarks underscore the fact that the line we draw between nature and culture is context-specific: to define a practice or behaviour as natural (organic, normative) or unnatural (artificial, perverse) is to make an ideological move.

The mobilisation of the nature–culture opposition has had an additional impact in relation to pregnancy. The concern to construct pregnancy as 'natural' can clearly be linked with the conventional assignation of woman to the sphere of nature and man to that of culture. In relation to the management of pregnancy, a recourse to 'nature' can, on occasion, work to women's practical advantage.

However, in the longer term, the construction of the pregnant woman as 'natural' serves to align her with the bodily and undermine her status as rational subject and social agent. Thus the influential nineteenth-century philosopher Herbert Spencer argued that woman's procreative function was incompatible with intellectual development: all the energy of women was needed for the reproductive process. He suggested that the physical and psychical differences between men and women had resulted from 'a somewhat earlier arrest of individual evolution in women than in men; necessitated by the reservation of vital power to meet the cost of reproduction'.[28] Such a view has obvious implications for the treatment of (pregnant) women. More recently, the feminist psychoanalyst Julia Kristeva, whose essay 'Stabat Mater' offers the most sophisticated of twentieth-century meditations on pregnancy, also seems to assimilate pregnancy to the natural and pre-cultural, of which we cannot be fully conscious. In her account of pregnancy, the mother's identity as a speaking subject is threatened by the splitting of her body and by reproductive processes over which she has no control:

> Cells fuse, split, and proliferate; volumes grow, tissues stretch, and body fluids change rhythm, speeding up or slowing down. Within the body, growing as a graft, indomitable, there is an other. And no one is present within that simultaneously dual and alien space, to signify what is going on. 'It happens, but I'm not there.' 'I cannot realize it, but it goes on.'[29]

Separating physiology and psychology, body and mind, Kristeva risks casting pregnancy in all too familiar terms as the surrender of woman's subject identity to the mysterious forces of nature.

None the less, the issues raised in 'Stabat Mater' are critical to an understanding of the subjective experience of pregnancy. What troubles the speaking 'I' in the passage quoted above is the presence within her body of 'an other' which 'she' cannot know. In 'The Ego and the Id', Freud argued that 'the ego is first and foremost a bodily ego'. In a footnote, his translator, James Strachey, added that 'the ego is ultimately derived from bodily sensations, chiefly from those springing from the surface of the body. It may thus be regarded as a mental projection of the surface of the body'.[30] Freud's concept of the bodily ego has been elaborated in a number of ways, most notably in Jacques Lacan's notion of the projected visual image of the body, and in Didier Anzieu's contrasting idea of the 'skin ego'.[31] What these perspectives share is the view that the bodily ego subtends and creates our sense of individual identity. What Freud calls 'the idea of our body', whether constructed primarily in visual terms or in terms of touch and sensation, founds our sense of the integrity of our individual existence. Pregnancy threatens to shatter this 'idea of the body'. As the pregnant body develops and grows, the visual image which the woman sees in the mirror no longer coincides with her internalised image of herself. At the same time, her 'bodily sensations', whether derived from the surface or depth of the body, are unfamiliar and disconcerting: they do not coincide with her previous knowledge of her body. Of course, such disturbances, and the threat to identity which they bring, characterise other physical conditions, particularly in cases where parts of the body are radically altered or removed. What is distinctive about pregnancy is the fact that the bodily space which we are accustomed to think of as our own is invaded by an other to whom we must attribute some degree of sentience, and hence individuality. Yet the border between the self and that other is never clear-cut: even the child's movements, evidence of its independence, are experienced as one's own. Hence Kristeva's description of the space of pregnancy as uninhabited ('no one is present'), 'dual and alien'. Within this space, the mother's identity has broken down: her body does not coincide with her idea of it, nor is it experienced as securely hers.

Kristeva's use of the word 'alien' is also striking, pointing to a sense of pregnancy as, paradoxically, both natural and monstrous. Descriptions of monstrous births were common in eighteenth- and nineteenth-century medical texts, and fear of such births has also been explored in many nineteenth- and twentieth-century literary texts and more recently in films such as *Rosemary's Baby* and *Alien*. Such fears are obviously connected on one level with simple uncertainty over the outcome of pregnancy. However, they can also be linked with a more general fear of the unknown, which in many cultures has found a focus (or scapegoat) in the figure of the pregnant woman. Mary Douglas has described the ways in which such fear finds expression in the taboos which surround pregnancy in many cultures. She writes of the liminal figure of the unborn child: '[i]ts present position is ambiguous, equally its future. For no one can say what sex it will have or whether it will survive the hazards of infancy. It is often treated as both vulnerable and dangerous.' She goes on to describe the way in which, when pregnant, 'a Lele woman tries to be considerate about not approaching sick persons lest the proximity of the child in her womb causes coughing or fever to increase'.[32] While much has been written about the taboos which surrounded pregnancy in Britain in the past, they have been interpreted almost exclusively in sexual terms. It is worth emphasising by contrast the complexity of these taboos, which were connected not only with the embarrassment inspired by visible signs of female sexual activity, but also with the fact that the pregnant body acts as both a reminder of our material origins and a signifier of the (uncertain) future.

This study takes the mid-eighteenth century as its starting point because this was a period in which the development of obstetrics (and the rise of the related disciplines of physiology and biology) revolutionised the understanding of pregnancy. The rise of obstetrics is linked with the increasing predominance of the 'man-midwife' in this period. As is well known, pregnancy and childbirth had previously been almost entirely under the control of women. Men were excluded from the delivery room, and surgeons were called in only as a last resort, to remove a dead foetus from the womb by craniotomy, for example (a practice whereby the skull was broken *in utero* in order that the foetus could be delivered). Towards the middle of the eighteenth century, however, medically qualified men began to turn their attention to the opportunities offered by this area of practice. It became common practice among the upper and middle classes to engage a man-midwife, or *accoucheur*, for childbirth: the fact that this was the established custom in France gave it a certain fashionable status. At the same time, because male practitioners who had become involved in this field had both the skills and the opportunities to undertake anatomical dissection, they were able to open up a new understanding of the processes of pregnancy and childbirth. In 1754, William Smellie published his *Anatomical Tables*, an obstetrical atlas which described for the first time the mechanisms of childbirth; in 1774, William Hunter published his *Anatomia Uteri Humani Gravidi (The Anatomy of the Human Gravid Uterus)*, which provided a detailed account of the development of the embryo/foetus and an explanation of the structure and function of the placenta. These obstetrical atlases were accompanied by treatises of midwifery which included Smellie's three-volume *A Treatise on the Theory and Practice of Midwifery* (1752–64), Alexander Hamilton's *A Treatise of Midwifery* (1781) and Thomas Denman's *An Introduction to the Practice of Midwifery* (1788). The new knowledge contained in these books was disseminated with relative rapidity, through well-attended lectures in schools of midwifery as well as through actual book sales.[33]

The understanding Smellie and Hunter were able to offer was grounded in anatomy but also, particularly in the case of Hunter, in knowledge of what we would now call physiology. Terminology was fluid in this period, and the terms physiology, biology and natural science were more or less interchangeable. However, the disciplines were emerging at this point in a more or less recognisably modern form, with an emphasis on the study of process rather than morphology in, respectively, human beings, animals and the natural world. An example of such work can be found in Erasmus Darwin's *Zoonomia: Or, The Laws of Organic Life* (1794), which set out to create a 'theory founded upon nature, that should bind together the scattered facts of medical knowledge, and converge into one point of view the laws of organic life'. Darwin argued that such a study was a necessary corrective to earlier, mechanistic attempts to understand the human body: rather than treating the body as 'an hydraulic machine' his approach involved 'comparing the properties belonging to animated nature with each other'.[34] Such an emphasis on comparative biology accorded with developments in contemporary medicine whereby older medical frameworks, in which disease was understood in terms of disequilibrium within the individual, were being supplanted by generic models of disease.

In Irvine Loudon's words, 'the eighteenth century was a period of phenomenal growth in obstetric knowledge, teaching and practice'. Advances in knowledge became widely available to practitioners through the textbooks on midwifery which appeared in growing numbers: as Loudon points out, 'the best of them, those by Smellie and especially Denman's works, were of astonishing maturity for their time'.[35] In addition, increased numbers of 'advice books' were published – texts on pregnancy written for the non-specialist reader by midwives and *accoucheurs*. These are among the diverse range of sources explored in chapter 1, which investigates the 'horizon of expectation' surrounding and inflecting the experience of pregnancy between 1750 and 1820.

1
Advice to the Fair Sex

Speaking of pregnancy: competing truth-claims

There have been several historical studies of the emergence of the
man-midwife, or *accoucheur*, in the eighteenth century and of the
gradual supplanting of the female midwife, first in upper-class and
then in middle-class households.[1] However, the main focus of such
accounts has been the struggle over the management of childbirth
and the use – and alleged abuse – of obstetric instruments. The
debate between midwives and *accoucheurs* over the management of
pregnancy has received less attention. This debate involved not only
practice, but also hermeneutics: indeed, the key issues were epistemological. How could pregnancy be known, and who had the authority
to speak of it? One of the fiercest exchanges in this respect was
between William Smellie and Elizabeth Nihell. The picture is interestingly complicated here in that the quarrel took place, at least in part,
by proxy. Elizabeth Nihell's *Treatise on the Art of Midwifery* was
thought by many to have been written by her husband, while Smellie
was defended against Nihell's attacks by his friend Tobias Smollett.
Smellie published the first two volumes of his *Treatise on the Theory
and Practice of Midwifery* in 1752 and 1754: these, like his *Anatomical
Tables* (1754), concentrated on an 'accurate' description of 'the situation of the parts concerned in parturition' and also gave practical
advice on 'touching' to diagnose pregnancy.

Nihell's response was vehement: her 1760 *Treatise* characterises the
activities of all man-midwives as gross and indelicate. In a swipe at
Smellie's anatomical background, she argued that many men-midwives
turned to midwifery because they were failed physicians, and she

considered with horror the prospect of a man-midwife's touching a woman:

> Will the husband be present? What must be the wife's confusion during so nauseous and so gross a scene? Will he *modestly* withdraw while his wife is so *served*? What must be his wife's danger from one of those rummagers, if she should be handsome enough to deserve his attention, or a compliment from him on such a visitation of her secret charms?[2]

Nihell deploys the coarse language of seduction ('served', 'rummagers') to depict an inappropriate invasion of female space. A contemporary engraving, 'The Man-midwife, or Female Delicacy after Marriage', is even more emphatic about the dangers of such encounters: the man-midwife examines a pregnant woman who lies in a seductive pose with one arm draped around him, as her husband is led out through a door surmounted by a picture of an ass (signifying cuckoldry). The pregnant woman is presented here as sexually attractive *and* active, in marked contrast with nineteenth-century representations of her as a quasi-virginal figure, removed from the sphere of sexual activity.[3] This understanding of the pregnant woman as an object of lustful desire is repeated in literary texts such as Charlotte Smith's *Montalbert*, although no indication is given there that the woman reciprocates such feelings.

Moving on from questions of modesty, and drawing on contemporary notions of 'consent' between parts of the body, Nihell argues that women practitioners have, by definition, a more finely tuned understanding of pregnancy. She writes that 'midwives, besides their personal experience, being sometimes themselves the mothers of children, have a kind of intuitive guide within themselves, the original organ of conception, itself pregnant, in more cases than that, with a strong instinctive influence on the mind and actions of the sex' (pp. 98–9). Despite her use of the term, Nihell's text is not simply invoking what we would now derogatively call 'female intuition'. The doctrine of consent proposed that organs or parts of the body were, under certain circumstances, in sympathy with each other. Pregnancy was a prime example, when it was thought that the excitation of the uterus after conception stimulated and disturbed the stomach and breasts. Alexander Hamilton, Professor of Midwifery at Edinburgh University, went so far as to argue in his 1781 *Treatise of Midwifery* that 'every part of the female frame sympathises with the womb'.[4] Moreover, the

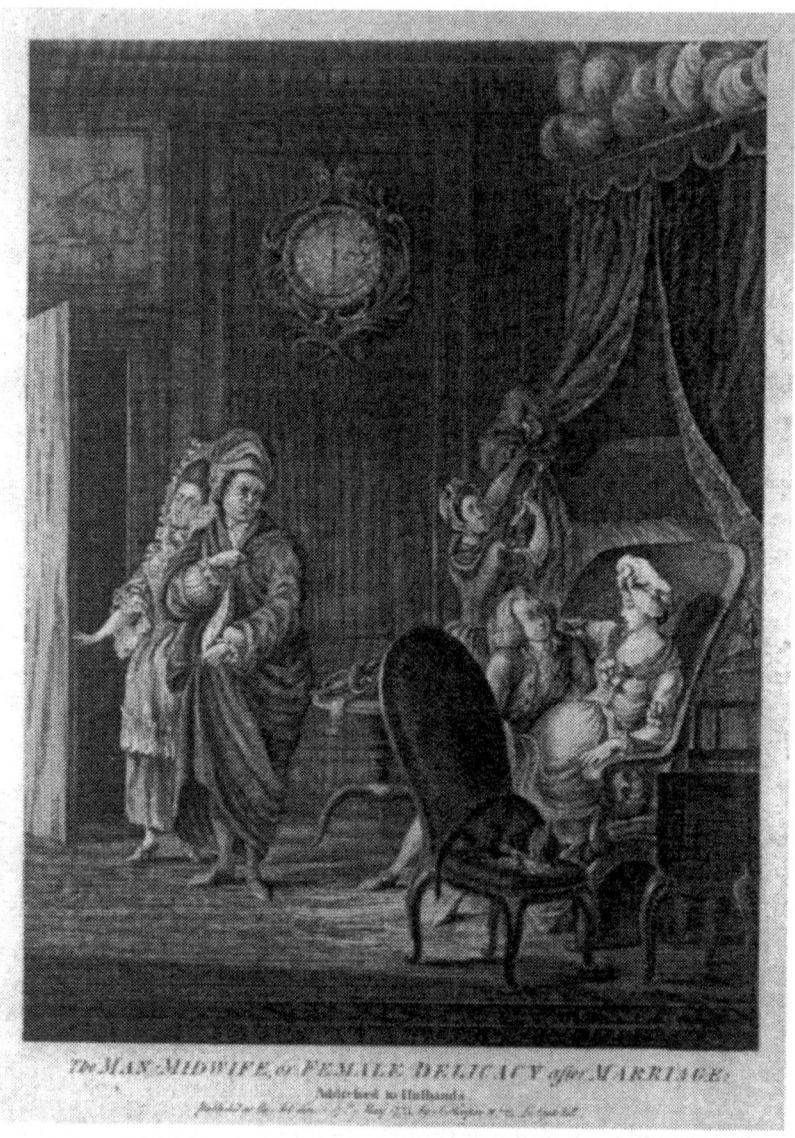

The MAN-MIDWIFE or FEMALE DELICACY after MARRIAGE.
Addressed to Husbands.

Figure 1   A male-midwife suggestively examines an attractive pregnant woman.
Line engraving, 1773. Wellcome Library, London.

notion of consent assumed, on occasion, a reciprocal influence
between mind and body. Nihell thus draws on an established school of
medical thought to ground her claim that female embodiment brought
sex-specific sensations and perceptions.

Smollett naturally took an entirely different line. Arguing in defence of Smellie in *The Critical Review*, he commented caustically that:

> the difference ... between the male-practitioner who has attended lectures, and the female who has not, is this; the first understands the animal oeconomy, the structure of the human body, the cure of distempers, the art of surgery, together with the theory and practice of midwifery, learned from the observations of an experienced artist, and the advantage of repeated delivery: the last is totally ignorant of everything but what she may have heard from an ignorant nurse or midwife, or seen at the few labours she has attended.[5]

The disagreement turned on the relative value of knowledge gained through sympathy versus observation. Nihell was arguing not only for the medical attendant's need to know the individual constitution of the patient, but also for a kind of sympathetic identification with their experience. Smollett, who had trained in medicine at Edinburgh, and who had assisted in the production of Smellie's *Treatise on the Theory and Practice of Midwifery*, was arguing for the superior diagnostic power of knowledge grounded in experimental physiology and in anatomy. Such knowledge was, of course, more readily available to male practitioners, but it was not unavailable to women: Smellie's classes, for example, were open to midwives. Nihell's appeal to the value of sympathetic experience *only* available to women was thus above all strategic, a political move in the struggle for control over obstetrics.

The struggle was intense because the stakes were relatively high. Attendance on a wealthy woman could be extremely lucrative for a qualified physician, who could charge far more than a midwife.[6] Yet it would be inaccurate to see the rise of obstetrics simply in terms of a movement driven by ambitious men who were able to exploit vulnerable female patients. The role of *accoucheur* certainly did offer a measure of upward social mobility. Thomas Denman, for example, was born in quite humble circumstances, as was William Hunter: both gradually built up extensive private practices among the aristocracy, and Hunter eventually became Physician-Extraordinary to Queen Charlotte.[7] Yet all the evidence would suggest that the rise of the *accoucheur* was achieved not through exploitation of women but in collaboration with them. The man-midwife could offer women a certain degree of protection by virtue of his professional status and women were not slow to perceive the advantages of this. For example, the authority of the *accoucheur* could be invoked in support of travel to (or indeed from) a husband or mother during pregnancy and confinement. The attendance of the *accoucheur* also added to the status of the pregnant woman: it added value to what might be called the profession of pregnancy among well-off women. The specialism of obstetrics thus emerged through a process of negotiation in which women were active participants, not passive dupes. Adrian Wilson makes a similar point in his study of man-midwives, but while he emphasises the role of the *accoucheur* as fashion statement (the employment of the man-midwife as 'conspicuous consumption', in his phrase), I would stress the role of the *accoucheur* as social protector. In this respect, it is significant that William Hunter staked out his claim to primacy in obstetrics on the basis of his understanding of women rather than on his (unparalleled) anatomical knowledge. In a paper on infanticide read to the Medical Society after his death in 1783, he wrote:

> The world will give me credit, surely, for having had sufficient opportunities of knowing a good deal of female characters. I have seen the private as well as the public virtues, the private as well as the more public frailties of women in all ranks of life. I have been in their secrets, their counsellor and adviser in the moments of their greatest distress in body and mind. I have been a witness to their private conduct, when they were preparing themselves to meet danger, and have heard their last and most serious reflections, when they were certain they had but few hours to live.[8]

Hunter's testimony, which also became his last testament, confirms the social, even psychological, role of the *accoucheur*. For although anatomical knowledge had increased rapidly over the previous twenty-five years, and Smellie, in particular, had shed new light on the processes of labour, many of the mechanisms of pregnancy and childbirth were still little understood. Most crucially, there was no means of monitoring foetal growth and development during pregnancy. It was not until 1822 that the foetal heartbeat was detected, opening up the possibility of auscultation to establish whether or not a foetus was alive.[9] While mechanical intervention in childbirth could save lives, for example through the use of forceps, in relation to pregnancy the function of the medical adviser remained overwhelmingly that of providing reassurance – antenatal care as placebo, so to speak. This is clear from a study of the advice books written by doctors in this period and aimed at female patients as adjuncts to or substitutes for personal consultation. Alexander Hamilton, for example, in his *Treatise on Midwifery* (written, according to him, in 'the most plain and familiar manner'), assures his readers 'that the pregnant state, however inconvenient, is generally free from other disorders; and that labour, though painful, is almost always natural, and the event happy' (p. xxiv). Repeatedly, women are urged to trust themselves to nature: so Denman confirms that 'in every thing which relates to the act of parturition Nature, not disturbed by disease, and unmolested by interruption, is fully competent to accomplish her own purpose'.[10] However, as has been noted in the Introduction, 'nature' is a slippery ideological construction. Here, in a paradox which continued to structure antenatal care, the authoritative professionals can do little more than suggest faith in nature, that is, *non*-intervention, as a medical strategy. Other than this, the advice in these texts consisted of bland injunctions to eat a balanced diet and exercise moderately. Venesection (blood-letting) was still sometimes recommended, and much attention was paid to constipation.[11] This latter was considered a serious matter, as it might lead women to use strong purgatives, which could in turn induce a miscarriage.

The medical profession found their lack of firm knowledge about pregnancy both frustrating and embarrassing, however. A telling case in this respect is that of Joanna Southcott, a self-educated prophet and visionary who achieved a cult following after she joined the Wesleyans in 1791. A year later she issued a series of 'sealed' prophesies and, in 1801, published a collection of writings, *The Strange Effects of Faith*. She eventually gained about 140,000 followers who formed an influential millenarian movement. In 1802 she predicted she would give birth to Shiloh, the second Christ, and in 1814, when she was 64, a 'miraculous' pregnancy was announced. In August of that year several doctors were called in to examine her, with conflicting results. Dr Richard Reece, author of the popular *Domestic Medical Guide* (1805), found her breasts enlarged and her abdomen distended. His account continues:

> These facts not being sufficient evidence of the pregnancy, I expressed a wish to be permitted to keep my right hand over the womb, for the purpose of discovering the motion of the foetus, on which she observed that it generally moved when she took nourishment; a piece of ripe fruit was then handed to her by her female attendant, on masticating which the motion of the foetus was very evident.

Reece was satisfied that she was pregnant.[12]

Dr John Sims, visiting on the same day, disagreed, finding her breasts plump only with 'the corpulence of an old woman' and detecting no foetal movement. He wished it to be put on record, however, that he

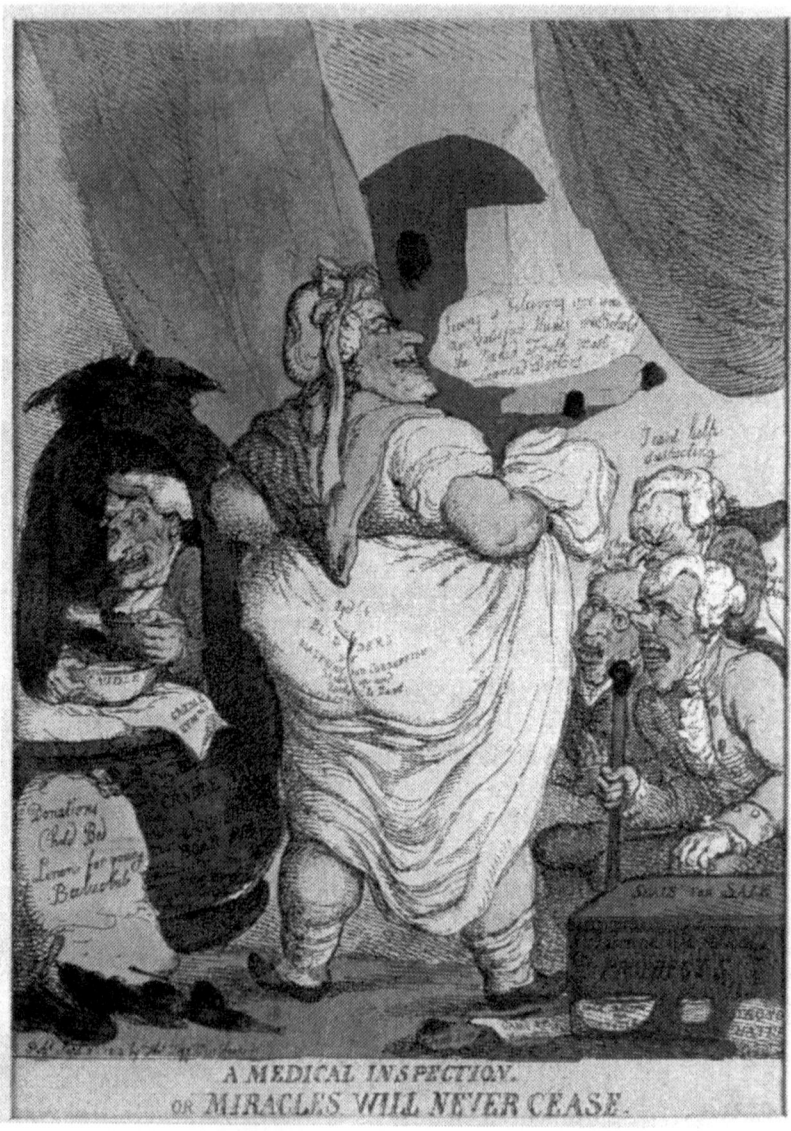

Figure 2   Joanna Southcott the prophetess exposing herself to three physicians
in order to validate her pregnancy. Coloured etching by T. Rowlandson, 1814.
Wellcome Library, London.

was convinced that 'this poor woman is no imposter, but that she labours under a strong mental delusion' (p. 27). Southcott continued to affirm her pregnancy, but acknowledged that 'should it prove not to be a child in the end, it must bring me to the grave'. She died on 27 December 1814 and, according to the *Dictionary of National Biography*, the autopsy revealed no pregnancy and no functional disorder or organic disease. However, in his 1837 *Exposition of the Signs and Symptoms of Pregnancy*, W.F. Montgomery claims that at the autopsy putrid matter was discovered, which did suggest disease. It is impossible to determine whether Southcott was in fact suffering from organic disease (for example, a tumour or fibroid growth) or whether hers was a case of what we would now call hysterical pregnancy.

The case became notorious and inspired much satirical comment, not only at the expense of Southcott but also at that of the clergymen and doctors who had supported her case. Thomas Rowlandson's cartoon 'A Medical Inspection: or Miracles Will Never Cease' is particularly instructive. It shows a monstrously corpulent Southcott, from the rear, lifting her skirts to display her belly and towering over a clergyman on her left and three doctors on her right. The clergyman is William Tozer, one of her staunchest followers: he crouches in her shadow drinking caudle (a spiced drink often administered to women to induce labour). The credulous doctors crouch on their knees next to a box labelled 'prophesies': the sketch suggests that their professional opinions are likely to be as fantastic and as little founded in fact as Southcott's prophesies. The case certainly fuelled public scepticism about the diagnostic powers of male practitioners, and Montgomery was still fuming about it twenty years later. In his monograph on the signs of pregnancy he refers repeatedly to Southcott the 'mock prophetess', accusing her of deliberate imposture and of manipulating her abdominal muscles in order to imitate foetal movements.[13]

Between 1750 and 1820, textbooks by *accoucheurs* increased rapidly in number, as the discourse of obstetric medicine became established. The sections which follow trace the dominant themes which are threaded through obstetric textbooks, advice books, medico-social and literary texts of the period, constructing a particular, if sometimes contradictory, cultural understanding of pregnancy.

Irritability/sensibility and maternal impressions

The physiological changes which take place in pregnancy were understood at this time primarily in terms of 'irritability', a term which, when applied to organs of the body, denoted an excessively or morbidly excitable condition. It was believed that the event of conception stimulated the womb, creating an excitability which in turn affected other organs which were in 'consent' (sympathy) with it. Thus Thomas Denman writes that 'the truth of no observation in medicine has been more generally acknowledged that that of the extreme irritability of the *uterus*, and of the propensity which the whole body has to be affected or disturbed by its influence' (p. 238). He goes on to explain that consent between the uterus and the breasts is 'intimate and constant' and it is this that causes the swelling of the breasts in pregnancy. The consent between the uterus and the stomach is also 'peculiarly frequent', hence the nausea of early pregnancy (pp. 239–40). Moreover, according to Denman and other authorities, there is a certain degree of 'consent' between the uterus and the mind or emotions:

> the whole habit of the body may be disturbed by a certain state of the *uterus*, and yet no individual part be peculiarly affected ... In consequence also of this general and perpetual irritation, the temper of pregnant women is sometimes rendered less gentle and patient than is consistent with their usual character. (p. 241)

We can detect here one of the seeds of that reworking of the Greek theory of the 'wandering womb' which was to support nineteenth-century discourses of female insanity. Indeed, some of Denman's contemporaries explicitly affirm that the 'irritability' of the uterus in pregnancy can lead to states of despondency bordering on insanity. John Grigg avers that 'throughout the whole period of pregnancy, women are more or less liable to dejection of spirits, hysteric affections, and sometimes to actual fainting' (p. 103) and Alexander Hamilton classes fainting and 'nervous or hysteric fits' among the disorders of pregnancy (p. 117). Martha Mears is the only writer who attempts to counter such negative views of irritability. In her determinedly upbeat *Candid Advice to the Fair Sex*, she describes pregnancy in glowing terms as a state of healthful fruition and takes issue with the very term 'irritability', asking:

> Is woman the only part of animated nature, whose powers are said to be weakened when she wants most to exert them; and who must pass, as it were, through the shades of death, to give life and nutriment to another being? Away with such a silly, such an impious idea ... Those

changes, which most pregnant women soon experience, are happily designed as notices of their situation, not as symptoms of infirmity. *What physicians term irritability, at that time, is but an increased sensibility of the womb, after it has received its precious deposit.*[14]

The sense of sensibility here is, however, ambiguous. For contemporary physiologists, 'sensibility' denoted the responsiveness of the nervous fibres to painful stimuli.[15] It may be that it is in this sense alone that Mears wishes to argue that the womb after conception is 'sensible', that is, responsive and alert to potential pain or danger, rather than morbidly irritable. However, whether intentionally or not, her use of the term invokes the contemporary cult of sensibility, meaning a capacity for emotional sensitivity and delicate feeling. Sensibility in this sense was closely bound up with the ideology of femininity and thus had a double-edged quality: while it implied that women in particular were capable of elevated and refined feeling, it also risked identifying them with feeling and sensation as opposed to reason.

Candid Advice to the Fair Sex is not a treatise on midwifery but an advice text aimed at a non-specialist female audience and with a very definite political and ideological purpose. As a midwife who is, she emphasises, herself a mother, Mears invokes the rhetoric of nature in order to resist the medicalisation of pregnancy associated with the rise of obstetrics. She describes the preparation of young women for their 'great purpose' of reproduction in florid terms: they develop 'rosy health' and 'a thousand new charms' as they anticipate 'the joy of becoming a mother'. As such language suggests, for Mears pregnancy is emphatically not a pathological condition. She argues that the state of pregnancy 'has too generally been considered as a state of indisposition or disease: this is a fatal error and the source of almost all the evils to which women in childbearing are liable' (p. 4). Mears also endorses the notion of sympathetic consent between mother and foetus, for this too supports her ideological project. Such an elaboration of the idea of consent is founded on the assumption that mother and foetus constitute *one body*, and this is a crucial move, for it implies that the mother has a privileged (sensational) knowledge of pregnancy, which cannot be available to the external observer. This takes us back to the epistemological problems posed by pregnancy. Mears wishes to fold the experience and knowledge of pregnancy back into the subjectivity of the mother because such maternal authority shores up, by extension, that of her female attendants.

Mears' polemical purpose is clear when she writes that it is 'the moderns' (i.e. male practitioners) who

> deny any mysterious consent between the mother and the *foetus*, because it cannot be explained on mechanical principles. Will they for the same reason deny the reciprocal influence of the mind and body? Would it be arguing like a physician or anatomist to deny the absorbing and filtering powers of the *placenta*, that medium of intercourse between the mother and child, because our dissecting instruments have not been able to trace, nor our glasses to discover to us in that organ either lymphatics or glands for performing such wonderful operations? (p. 57)

The effect of Mears' stance is ambiguous, however. On the one hand, in endorsing maternal authority, she helps to sustain the mother as the proper subject, or agent, of pregnancy. On the other, in using the terminology of sensibility and 'mysterious' consent, she risks aligning the maternal with feeling rather than thought.[16]

The notion of maternal impressions was closely related to ideas of irritability (or sensibility) and of consent between mother and foetus. The idea that a pregnant woman's imagination could affect her unborn child, creating marks and deformities, was a longstanding folk belief which, as Philip Wilson has shown, was taken up into medical discourse in the eighteenth century.[17] In 1727 James Blondel published anonymously a pamphlet titled 'The Strength of Imagination in Pregnant Women Examined', which sought to refute the idea on rational grounds. Blondel argued that, while it was undoubtedly true that physical accidents or emotional distress could bring on miscarriage, many women suffered such events without any adverse effect: similarly, many mothers of marked or deformed children had experienced entirely calm and peaceful pregnancies. Blondel's paper provoked an immediate response from Daniel Turner, who strongly defended the idea (which he had earlier utilised in his 1714 book on skin disease) that the mother's imagination could make a physical impression on the malleable foetus. The dispute drew a considerable amount of attention: two more pamphlets followed from Blondel and Turner and provoked several interventions by others. Those who supported the idea of maternal impressions thought that the mother's imagination could be so strongly affected by longing or loathing for particular objects that the physical form of these objects could be imprinted on the developing embryo/foetus. However, the consensus among man-midwives/obstetricians by the late eighteenth century was against a belief in maternal impressions in such a literal sense, however beguiling stories about them might be. Smellie, for example, was much taken by a story of maternal longing from one of his patients, who had on the tip of her tongue something like a plum 'of a green colour', which was hard and painful:

> She told me that when plumbs [*sic*] begin to ripen, it grows larger, softer and less painful, acquires a blue, reddish or purple colour, and she feels a hard grisly substance like the stone in the middle: in winter it shrivels and decreases, and next season resumes the same appearance. It seems when her mother was with child of her, she longed for some plumbs, which she cheapned, but would not buy, because she thought them too dear; however, she had touched the tip of her tongue with one of them, which she afterwards threw down, and by this transient touch the child was affected in the same place.[18]

None the less, Smellie was sceptical of the effect of thwarted longings or cravings on the developing child. Equally, he resisted the idea that disagreeable impressions could affect the child: he pointed out that he had delivered many children who had retained no marks even though their mothers were 'frightened and surprized by disagreeable objects' and feared the consequences of such impressions (p. 210). Grigg offered similar arguments, and recommended pregnant women not to listen 'to the idle stories of gossips' (p. 121). Erasmus Darwin was characteristically wayward in supporting the notion of impressions – but in his case, it was *paternal* impressions. In *Zoonomia* he argued that the world had 'long been mistaken in ascribing great power to the imagination of the female' and that 'the real power of imagination, in the act of gestation, belongs solely to the male'.[19] According to him, the image in the mind of the father at the time of copulation, or at the time of the secretion of the semen, 'may so affect this secretion by irritative or sensitive association ... as to cause the production of similarity of form and of features, with the distinction of sex'. The notion that paternal impressions were responsible for the child's sex involved Darwin in somewhat convoluted explanations to account for why the father would be thinking of a male form during the act of coition.[20]

Although *accoucheurs* and professors of midwifery doubted the power of the imagination to make a literal mark on the developing child, they were in agreement about the potentially dangerous effects of excessive emotion in pregnancy. Hamilton warned against 'crowds, confinement, every situation which renders [pregnant women] under any disagreeable restriction ... and whatever disturbs either the body or mind' (p. 161); and Grigg explained that miscarriage could arise from 'the indulgence of violent passions, a mode of living inconsistent with the order and simplicity of nature, a view of objects in distress or in imminent danger, the hearing of dreadful accounts, or reading melancholy stories, in short, whatever else can either injure the body or disturb the mind' (pp. 117–18). Harrowing case histories were related of miscarriage or stillbirth in such circumstances, and the mother's responsibility for a healthy pregnancy was emphasised. The professional politics of such insistence are complex. Obstetrics, like other emerging medical specialisms, was grounded in rational enquiry and empirical observation: hence scepticism among male *accoucheurs* about 'maternal impressions' in the literal sense. However, the strongly held belief in the effect of the mother's emotions on the health of the unborn child was *not* securely grounded in reason or empirical observation, which suggest that it must be viewed primarily as an ideological construction, bound up with contemporary cultural imperatives. While the older belief in maternal impressions reflected a sense of the almost uncanny power of the pregnant woman (who none the less could not be held responsible for the impressions she received), the new emphasis was on the need for the pregnant woman to control her emotional state. This more sophisticated doctrine of maternal impressions might better be called one of maternal responsibility, for it encouraged women to internalise the medico-social view of their responsibility for pregnancy and, in consequence, to discipline their emotions and adopt 'appropriate' (constrained) behaviour. By a curious cultural sleight of hand, knowledge about the effect of maternal impressions was transferred to the male practitioner, whereas responsibility for such impressions (and for the medical outcome) was assigned to the pregnant woman.

In this context, it is perhaps not surprising that maternal responsibility should form a recurrent, even obsessive, theme in women's writing of this period. The case of Mary Wollstonecraft is instructive in this as in so many other respects. In *A Vindication of the Rights of Woman*, published in 1792, she had argued bravely that women should act as rational creatures, 'despising that weak elegancy of mind, exquisite sensibility, and sweet docility of manners, supposed to be the sexual characteristics of the weaker vessel'.[21] None the less, when a year later she became involved with Gilbert Imlay and subsequently became pregnant with his child, she wrote miserably to him of what she saw as her own frequent yielding to sensibility and failure to control her emotions in pregnancy:

> It is time for me to grow *more reasonable*, a few more of these *caprices of sensibility* would destroy me. I have, in fact, been very much indisposed for a few days past, and the notion that I was torment-ing, or perhaps killing, a poor little animal, about whom I am grown anxious and tender, now I feel it alive, made me worse.[22]

Three days later, referring to the fact that she had allowed herself to be upset by Imlay's coldness to her, she wrote that she had been 'seriously alarmed and angry with myself, dreading continually the fatal conse-quence of my folly' (p. 245). As the violence of her language suggests, Wollstonecraft feels herself almost a murderer: her initial distress over Imlay is compounded by the fear that her emotional reactions may be damaging her child. She was not in a position to contest prevailing medical views about the effect of emotion on her unborn child, and the result was a wearing degree of self-blame.

None the less, although Wollstonecraft and her contemporaries did not question the facts of maternal responsibility (i.e. the proposition that maternal emotions could affect the health of the developing child), they deployed the concept in their fiction to interrogate the contexts of such responsibility. Their fiction thus foregrounds the con-ditions under which a pregnant woman might come to suffer 'exces-sive' emotion, and often depicts the situation of the pregnant woman as an extreme case of the social and legal exploitation of all women. While women could at this time, exceptionally, have their property protected for their own use under the system of equity, the provisions of common law entailed the loss of a woman's legal identity upon marriage. Women were in effect exchanged as property between fathers and husbands, and one of their prime functions was to act as conduits for inheritance. Hence the emphasis on women's chastity to ensure that the line of inheritance was secured for legitimate sons.

Wollstonecraft's unfinished novel *Maria* focuses sharply on this issue. Maria has been married against her will to a brutish and dissi-pated husband, who steadily spends the money for which he has married her. Soon after she becomes pregnant, she discovers that he has been encouraging another man to have an affair with her in the hope of securing a necessary loan. She resolves to leave, but in order to keep this resolution Wollstonecraft suggests, significantly, that she has to 'disengage' mind and body, as though to act as a rational creature were incompatible with pregnant embodiment. After her successful escape, however, mind and body collapse back into each other, with the result that she begins to fear for the child who is coterminous with her body and who will, she assumes, be affected by her state of mind:

> My mind, during the few past days, seemed, as it were, disengaged from my body; but, now the struggle was over, I felt very forcibly the effect which perturbation of spirits produces on a woman in my situation.
>
> The apprehension of a miscarriage, obliged me to confine myself to my apartment near a fortnight.[23]

It is clear that it is her husband's brutal treatment which has caused Maria's 'perturbation of spirits', and that this brutal treatment is grounded in a legal system which makes a wife, in Maria's vivid phrase, 'as much a man's property as his horse, or his ass' (p. 118). This is further underscored when Maria's uncle dies at the same time that her daughter is born, leaving his property to the daughter, with Maria as guardian. By this means he hoped to enable Maria 'to be mistress of his fortune, without putting any part of it in [her husband's] power'. This plan is to no avail, however. In (re)producing a daughter, Maria has provided another piece of valuable property for her husband, who manages to abduct the child and then confines Maria to a lunatic asylum. Despite these rather Gothic plot embellishments, the text reflects the reality of the fact that a woman in Maria's position would have had little redress against a husband who acted against her interests, but was still her primary legal protector.

If Wollstonecraft reworked aspects of her own experience in *Maria*, she also had the dubious privilege of having another novelist posthumously reworking the material of her life. Amelia Opie was a close friend whose novel *Adeline Mowbray, or The Mother and Daughter*, published in 1805, was allegedly based on the relationship between Wollstonecraft and her husband, William Godwin. *Adeline Mowbray* has been seen as an attack on the free-thinking, Godwinian view of marriage and as part of the reaction against radical Jacobin ideas which characterised the post-revolutionary period. However, a consideration of the theme of maternal responsibility as it is explored in the novel shows that Opie, like Wollstonecraft, was prepared to engage critically with the social framework which conditioned women's feelings. The plot turns on a young woman who fails to realise that her mother's 'freethinking' beliefs are purely theoretical. When she naively puts her mother's ideas into practice, living openly with the young philosopher Glenmurray, whose books she has read and whose ideas she has imbibed, she is, unsurprisingly, rejected by both her mother and society. She defies public opinion until, after the death of Glenmurray, she realises her error of judgement and slowly makes her way back towards social acceptance. The idea of maternal responsibility is central to the novel and is explored on a number of interlocking levels. First, the freethinking Mrs Mowbray is shown to have failed her daughter through her irresponsible advocacy of theories she herself would never put into practice and which for her are simple 'amusements'. She further neglects her responsibilities when, as her friend Dr Norberry puts it, at the age of forty she plays the fool and marries 'a penniless profligate, merely because he had a fine person and a handsome leg': it is this second husband's attempted seduction of Adeline which prompts her elopement with Glenmurray. Third, Mrs Mowbray is duped by a relation who conceals Adeline's many letters asking for forgiveness. Her failure to ask what is going on and actively seek out her daughter contributes to Adeline's decline and eventual death.

It is through Adeline that the specificity of maternal responsibility in pregnancy is explored. Adeline's pregnancy occurs in the context of a union founded only on the ties of love and reason. She scorns conventional marriage and painstakingly defends her position against those who argue that her union is immoral in the eyes of God. Yet, although Adeline thinks that her position is founded on reason, she discovers too late that reason, unlike 'amusing' speculation, must take into account the 'world as it is' in formulating principles of behaviour. Seven months into her pregnancy, she sees some children playing on a terrace but excluding one boy from their game. When she asks why, she is told that he is a bastard and so is not fit company for the others. Adeline suffers and weeps with him, realising that this may be the fate of her own child:

> The cause of the child's affliction was a dagger in her heart; and, while she listened to the now redoubled sobs of the disgraced and proudly afflicted boy, she was driven almost to phrensy [sic]: for 'Such,' she exclaimed, 'may one time or other be the pangs of my child, and so to him may the hours of childhood be embittered!' – Again she seated herself by the little mourner – and her tears accompanied his.[24]

As the language suggests, Adeline's mental and physical torments are inextricably intertwined: her body speaks her feelings. The 'horror' she witnesses affects her so powerfully that she just has strength to return to Glenmurray and ask him to marry her, before she falls senseless to the floor. However, it is too late to avert the ill-effects of this 'maternal impression'. After a brief return to consciousness, Adeline relapses into a fainting fit, and the day after the encounter on the terrace gives birth to a dead child.

To an extent, this episode could have stepped straight out of a text-book of obstetrics as a warning of the dangers posed by unregulated emotion. It also seems to reflect dominant ideology in that Adeline's suffering is presented as the direct result of her sin. Had she not lived with Glenmurray outside marriage, her perception of danger and hence the death of the child would simply not have occurred. This point is reinforced by the fact that Adeline's second child, the product of the marriage she makes after Glenmurray's death, thrives ostentatiously, even surviving smallpox. Yet Opie's text opens up more than one contradiction and remains especially ambivalent over the question of marriage. Adeline is constructed as a character who is entirely virtuous and amiable, her only fault being her (principled) refusal to marry Glenmurray. The narrative perspective, foreground-ing the other characters' perception of Adeline as virtuous when she is thought to be married and vicious as soon as the truth is discov-ered, poses the question of the relationship between inherent or natural virtue and religious doctrine. Must Adeline's failure to marry be considered an absolute sin? It foregrounds, too, the pernicious effects of prejudice: as Adeline herself puts it: 'Because an idle cere-mony has not been muttered over me at the altar, I am liable to be thought a woman of vicious inclinations, and to be exposed to the most daring insults' (p. 116). And while the text finally endorses mar-riage as a 'hallowed institution', it restlessly returns to the question of the disproportion between Adeline's single crime (not marrying Glenmurray) and her multiple punishments (the death of her child, social ostracism, poverty).

More disturbing is a thread which runs through many representa-tions of maternal impressions, not just in literary texts but in letters and textbooks of obstetrics. As we have seen, an emphasis on the effect of maternal emotions on the unborn child can all too easily slide into a construction of the mother as a creature of emotions, peculiarly susceptible to feeling because of her pregnant state. While the link between mother and foetus can be construed in such a way as to protect the authority and autonomy of pregnant women, it can equally be turned round to justify an argument for pregnant embodiment as implying potential loss of reason. Adeline's 'fits of phrensy' and 'paroxysms of sorrow' certainly support the construction of the pregnant woman as subject to, rather than author of, her emotions and attachments. The text might seem to suggest that in terms of maternal responsibility, Adeline's fault is having too much sensibility, while her mother's is having too little. Yet at the end of the novel, when Adeline is once again held in the loving gaze of her mother, maternal feeling is again powerfully endorsed:

> Mrs Mowbray at that moment eagerly and anxiously pressed forward to catch her weak accents, and inquire how she felt. 'I have seen that fond and anxious look before,' she faintly articulated, 'but in happier times! and it assures me that you love me still.'
>
> 'Love you still!' replied Mrs Mowbray with passionate fondness: – 'never, never were you so dear to me as now!' (p. 268)

To this extent, *Adeline Mowbray* offers a conservative and regressive version of the mother–daughter plot, which features in several novels of the period. Adeline wishes to return to the pre-Oedipal relationship between mother and daughter rather than continue to confront the injustices of society, and experiences her death in terms of a longed-for restoration to the asocial maternal body. By contrast, contemporary novels by Mary Hays and Charlotte Smith represent daughters who learn from the narratives and teachings of their self-critical mothers.[25] Charlotte Smith's *The Young Philosopher* (1798) is, like *Adeline Mowbray*, based in part on the lives of Godwin and Wollstonecraft: Loraine Fletcher suggests that the character of Armitage is based on Godwin, and that of Glenmorris on Tom Paine.[26] Smith's novel also resembles Wollstonecraft's *Maria* in its emphasis on the relationship between pregnancy and property. The novel explores the fate of Laura de Verdun and her daughter Medora, the first names of mother and daughter echoing each other closely. In the embedded narrative, we learn of the young Laura's falling in love with the freethinker Glenmorris and marrying him against her parents' will. After the marriage, they live happily on his rundown estate in Scotland. However, when Laura is pregnant, Glenmorris is attacked and captured and is so seriously injured that Laura believes he is dead. Her husband's only surviving relation, the aptly named Lady Kilbrodie, realising that Glenmorris's estate will pass to her son if Glenmorris's child does not survive, takes Laura to live with her with the sole aim of ensuring the death of the child.

While Lady Kilbrodie sees Laura's pregnancy clearly in its social context, with Laura as the channel for Glenmorris's inheritance, her means of attack is through the private and affective notion of maternal impressions. She seeks to instil fear and anxiety in Laura in the hope that this will bring about a miscarriage. Laura describes her attempts to terrify through the use of religious discourse and superstition:

> She ... talked to me of the judgments of heaven, which she said always pursued, and sooner or later overtook, undutiful children ... As the time of my lying-in approached, she caused the superstitions of the country to be brought forward, to alarm me with ideas of danger and dread of death.[27]

Smith emphasises the fact that, up to this point, Laura uses reason to resist the 'cant' of Lady Kilbrodie. However, she is unable to withstand the additional pressure when the son appears and embarks on detailed and bloodcurdling descriptions of the torture of military prisoners. As Glenmorris was taken by buccaneers, the effect on Laura's susceptible imagination is immediate:

> The barbarous wretch, seeing by the changes of my countenance, how unable I was to sustain the recital, proceeded to relate these scenes, so disgraceful to humanity, more minutely ... The terms he used, the wild contortions of his countenance, and the terrible idea, that, to the reality of what I could not bear to hear, Glenmorris might have been exposed, at length so far overcame me, that I could suffer no more. – A cold dew covered my face – I felt the room turn round with me, and fell totally insensible on the floor. (Vol. 2, pp. 117–18)

Particularly notable in this passage is a preoccupation with facial expression. Laura's distress is evident from the 'changes of her countenance'; her tormentor's effects are gained through 'the wild contortions of his countenance'; finally, before she swoons, Laura's face is covered by 'a cold dew'. It could be argued that the face is the primary site or surface on which the somatic effects of emotion are visible – hence Smith's emphasis. For it is at this point that Smith closes the loop of 'maternal impressions'. Laura's 'irritable' pregnant body has produced a susceptibility to emotion which in turn feeds back to damage the body. Her suffering brings on an early labour, which she has the strength to endure in secret without the ministrations of a midwife. However, her seven months' child is 'small and feeble' and although Laura wishes 'to preserve him, and to live for him, with an ardour amounting even to agony', the child falls into convulsions on the third day and dies in her arms.

Laura's narrative is in many respects in accord with contemporary obstetric narratives and follows them closely. In relation to her fears in pregnancy, for example, she notes that 'these presentiments of evil are often the causes that evil really arrives, especially to persons in my circumstances', echoing almost exactly William Buchan's words in the best-selling guide *Domestic Medicine*: 'The constant dread of some future evil, by dwelling upon the mind, often occasions the very evil itself ... This, for example, is often the case with women in childbed.'[28] However, where Smith diverges from medical narratives is in her insistence, not least through the flamboyant and melodramatic twists of her plot, on the social imbrication of pregnancy. Smith, like Opie, foregrounds the fact that maternal impressions are culturally as well as physiologically constructed, in this case as the nervousness of an unprotected woman is deliberately manipulated by those whose interests she threatens. In Laura's case the damage is permanent, not only because her son dies but because she never regains her earlier firmness of mind. In consequence when, many years later, her daughter Medora is abducted, Laura falls into a violent 'phrensy' and loses her reason: 'she shrieked aloud, called incessantly on her daughter, walked in a frantic manner round the room ... the agony of her mind became so great as to produce all the appearances of actual madness.'[29] Laura's maternal impressions lead to a permanent weakening of the intellect, and in this she is the precursor of various nineteenth-century fictional heroines who suffer from the 'insanity of pregnancy'. Yet through the character of Medora, Smith suggests that excess sensibility, with all its damaging effects, can and must be resisted. Medora learns from her mother's story, so that when she is threatened with rape she speaks up against her attackers, using the language of reason rather than of feeling to defend herself. While Laura is the victim of a 'too acute sensibility, too hastily indulged', Medora has a sensibility which is carefully distinguished by Smith from both that of her mother *and* that of the heroines of Gothic fiction. Smith writes: 'Her sensibility was not the exotic production of those forced and unnatural descriptions of tenderness, that are exhibited by the imaginary heroine of impossible adventures; it was the consequence of right and genuine feelings' (Vol. 3, p. 38).

To some extent we might read across from the distinction between Laura and Medora in Smith's novel and that between Marianne and Elinor in Jane Austen's *Sense and Sensibility*. In neither case is this distinction absolute or clear-cut: Laura and Marianne possess both acute feelings and a good understanding; Elinor and Medora possess sense and a sensibility grounded in 'right and genuine feelings'. However, there is another connection: *Sense and Sensibility* is the only Austen novel in which pregnancy receives more than a glancing reference. The fact that pregnancy should figure at all is perhaps not surprising in the context of contemporary ideas about the link between pregnancy and sensibility. *Sense and Sensibility* pairs a number of female characters, one of the most telling juxtapositions being that between Marianne and Mrs Palmer, whose stories run in counterpoint at one point in the novel. Mrs Palmer's narrative can be read in terms of the triumph of maternal *in*sensibility. She is, in Elinor's view, 'a very silly woman', not malicious but resistant to thought and introspection, cheerfully and determinedly brushing aside not only social embarrassments but her husband's contemptuous disregard for her. We learn of her pregnancy when she is first introduced to the Dashwoods and are updated on its progress though her mother's reports and enquiries: for example, Mrs Jennings asks Colonel Brandon when he has been dining at the Palmers, 'How do they all do at their house? How does Charlotte do? I warrant you she is a fine size by this time.'[30] Her pregnancy progresses without any difficulties and she is eventually delivered of a son and heir, an event which is 'very satisfactory' to all concerned. While Charlotte waxes, however, Marianne wanes. After Willoughby's rejection of her she descends into anorexia, which is described as a symptom of her 'nervous irritability' (p. 150). Her decline can be read as a kind of shadow or reverse-image of Mrs Palmer's pregnancy. As Maud Ellmann has pointed out, many anorexics see food and impregnation as identical, for each involves the invasion of the body and a violation of self-identity. Rejection of the one constitutes, in fantasy at least, rejection of the other.[31] Marianne can thus be read as a female figure whose 'irritability' works on this occasion to preclude pregnancy, on the level of fantasy and metaphor at least.

Austen also depicts Marianne as acting out her emotional distress in somatic and gestural ways. She writes, 'no attitude could give her ease; and in restless pain of mind and body she moved from one posture to another, till growing more and more hysterical, her sister could with difficulty keep her on the bed at all, and for some time was fearful of being constrained to call for assistance' (p. 159). The term 'hysterical' is significant. It is used here in the context of the new science of neurology and the understanding associated with it of the body as a network of nerves and fibres, vibrating with impressions and sensations. However, in the nineteenth century hysteria rapidly became identified with specifically female 'nervousness'. I would argue that the notions of maternal impressions and irritability/sensibility tied in with and helped to support this gendering of mental instability. For if it was accepted that the pregnant woman was rendered 'irritable' by uterine stimulation and hence susceptible to emotion, the corollary would be that all women of reproductive age would be similarly affected by uterine changes. Though the menstrual cycle was not well understood, the connection between ovulation and menstruation was recognised, as were periodical changes in the lining of the womb. It was thus possible to develop a specifically uterine 'causal' model for female instability, in the same way that a hormonal model could be developed and deployed in the twentieth century.

Valuing pregnancy

As a social function, reproduction is laden with social and economic meanings, and in this context some pregnancies are always considered more valuable, both economically and ideologically, than others. An examination of a range of texts from this period reveals two specific and related discourses which attempt to discriminate between 'good' and 'bad' pregnancies. The first is that of differential breeding, which is grounded in the fear that certain sections of the population are breeding more successfully than others and that this may destabilise the social order. In the late eighteenth and early nineteenth centuries, there was a widespread belief that the rural poor were breeding more successfully than any other class, while the aristocracy were failing to reproduce in adequate numbers. This 'fact' is presented as certainty by William Buchan in *Domestic Medicine*, in which he writes:

> It is very certain that high living vitiates the humours, and prevents fecundity. We seldom find a barren woman among the labouring poor, while nothing is more common amongst the rich and affluent ... Would the rich use the same sort of food and exercise as the better sort of peasants, they would seldom have cause to envy their poor vassals and dependents the blessing of a numerous and healthy offspring, while they pine in sorrow for the want of even a single heir to their extensive dominions. (p. 667)

His words are echoed in a different context in Adam Smith's 1776 *The Wealth of Nations*, in which it is claimed that 'a half-starved Highland woman frequently bears more than twenty children, while a pampered fine lady is often incapable of bearing any, and is generally exhausted by two or three. Barrenness, so frequent among women of fashion, is very rare among those of inferior station.'[32] Smith did not fear that this would bring about any change in the social order, however, but took the view that the high birth rate among the labouring classes would be offset by high infant mortality, and that labour levels and the class structure would thus remain stable.

It was the *accoucheurs*, not unnaturally, who were most concerned with the question of barrenness among the wealthy: this was, after all, the class on which their living depended. Nor is it surprising, in view of their lack of accurate knowledge of the processes of conception, that they should fall back again on 'nature' as the guarantor of fertility. Denman follows Buchan in linking an open-air life with reproductive success, and in warning against over-indulgence and 'high living'. He argues that:

> the lower class of women, who are by necessity obliged to follow laborious occupations in the open air, and who are exposed to all the vicissitudes of the weather, not only pass the time of their pregnancy with fewer complaints than the affluent, but have also more easy labours ...Those who are in possession of all the advantages of rank and fortune, which the eyes of inferiors are apt to look at with envy, must use them with the most cautious moderation, or they will suffer for every unreasonable indulgence. (p. 250)

Yet the belief that barrenness was common among the rich is not borne out by the evidence. The registration of live births dates only from 1837 in England and Wales, 1855 in Scotland and 1864 in Ireland, so we do not have an accurate record of the birth rate prior to this, nor of its relation to social class. However, studies of specific groups of upper- and middle-class women reveal relatively high birth rates. Lewis, for example, analysed a group of fifty aristocratic British women in the period 1760–1860. She found that the average span of their child-bearing years was eighteen and the average number of live children they bore eight. These women thus had high rates of fertility and productivity, despite the fears expressed over 'pampered ladies'.[33] Similarly, Davidoff and Hall's work on the provincial middle classes suggests an average child-bearing span of thirteen

years, and an average of seven children.[34] Actual fertility may have
been even higher, for as Angus McLaren has argued, fertility controlling strategies, including induced abortion, were resorted to by all
classes in this period.[35]

Although it is not possible to recover accurate statistics for the period
1750–1820, it is clear that the alleged contrast between aristocratic
barrenness and rustic fertility was mythical rather than actual. The dissemination of the myth in medical texts was probably driven by a
number of factors. For a handful of aristocratic families, there would
have been real concerns about barrenness because of the implications
for inheritance: such concerns had to be addressed in textbooks
written by *accoucheurs* like Denman. Also in play, however, were anxieties about the deleterious effects of luxurious urban life on all aspects
of health, not just fertility and safe delivery. Finally, there was an
implicit fear of the vitality of the rural poor which can be linked with
the revolutionary decade of the 1790s and with agrarian protests
against the Enclosure Acts. These led to the break-up of six million
acres of common land between 1760 and 1830, land on which many
rural workers depended for the tending of livestock and the gathering
of fuel. Men and women pulled down fences and gates in protest
against this threat to their livelihood. Some medical texts might well
have reflected and reinforced anxieties about such protest. Gradually,
however, as the rural population declined in percentage terms,
attention shifted to the condition of the urban poor. Their health came
under far more systematic scrutiny, particularly from doctors working
in the newly established hospitals and dispensaries. One such figure
was Augustus Bozzi Granville who, in 1818, published a report on the
practice of midwifery at the Westminster General Dispensary. He
argued that dispensaries were more acceptable to the poor than the
workhouse ('the very name of which causes distress to the feelings') or
the lying-in (that is, maternity) hospital, 'where [the woman] becomes
a conspicuous object of public charity'.[36] Moreover, Dispensary care
was cheap, as women were attended at home, and thus more women
could be helped: according to his calculations, the cost of one labour at
a lying-in hospital (£3 12s 10d) would support sixteen labours
associated with the Westminster.

Granville was a statistician who expressed with some trenchancy his
views on the supposed distinction in matters of health between women
who live a 'luxurious' life and those who live 'in a state of nature'.
Taking the test case of repeated miscarriage (then, as now, a particularly
distressing occurrence), he questioned and examined 'these supposed

privileged people – "the lower ranks of life"'. He concluded that, with regard to miscarriage, no privileged class exists: 'the majority of those causes to which the frequent occurrence of that event must necessarily be ascribed, act equally on the wretched inhabitants of the Seven-dials [an area of London notorious for its poverty and dereliction], and on the more fortunate inmates of a Palace' (p. 40).

The notion of the greater reproductive power of those who live in 'a state of nature' continued to feature in medical texts until well into the nineteenth century. W.F. Montgomery, for example, writing in 1837, attacked 'fine ladies, who lounge all day long on their sofa or spend half their day in bed, gratifying a mere indolence of habit which they calculate on being allowed or even encouraged to indulge in, on account of their situation'. Such inactivity, he claimed, threatened to induce a 'universal torpor' of the system. He went on to paint a contrasting picture of bucolic reproductive health: 'How different this from the joyous buoyancy of the sturdy peasant female, whose daily round of laborious occupations is continued without interruption to almost "the hour of nature's sorrow"' (p. 11). This emphasis on rural fecundity and fear of a falling birth rate among the upper classes can be read as a kind of proto-eugenics, paving the way for the development of eugenic thought associated with Francis Galton in the later nineteenth century.

The second discriminatory discourse is that of il/legitimacy, which is a regulatory structure as well as a discourse, with very real material effects. In the late eighteenth and early nineteenth centuries the relationship between pregnancy and the law was unstable and remains somewhat obscure. The effect of Lord Hardwicke's 1753 Marriage Act is particularly difficult to assess. Prior to the passing of the Act, the custom of betrothal among the lower classes had sanctioned sex before marriage, and indeed in some parts of Britain women were expected to 'prove' their fertility by becoming pregnant in the betrothal period.[37] The combination of social pressure and, if necessary, recourse to the church courts meant that such women were virtually guaranteed marriage. However, Hardwicke's Act stipulated that a marriage was legal only if vows were exchanged in a recognised place of worship after the calling of banns or the purchase of a licence. Under the terms of the new Act, a betrothal was no longer recognised as having a coercive or sanctioning power. Despite this, Nicholas Rogers has argued that poorer women continued to use their sexuality in order to secure marriage partners, deliberately getting pregnant and expecting marriage to follow. The statistics would suggest that this strategy was often successful: by the early nineteenth century about a third of brides were pregnant at the time of their marriage.[38] Equally, however, marriage did not always follow pregnancy, and illegitimacy rates also rose. In mid-eighteenth-century London, about 16 per cent of first births were illegitimate, and the rates continued to rise overall until the late nineteenth century.[39]

It was the rise in the illegitimacy rate which caused concern among all classes, although the form that such concern took varied according to class perspective and social status. It was recognised that for very poor women the birth of an illegitimate child could spell disaster, and the situation of such women was sympathetically treated by women writers and the medical profession. This was particularly true of those who worked in domestic service and who would be sacked as soon as their condition became known, particularly if the father were the master of the house. Mary Wollstonecraft's *Maria* explores such a situation through the character of the servant Jemima, born into abject poverty and effectively raped by her master when she is sixteen years old. Her emotions when she discovers she is pregnant are complex: she feels 'a mixed sensation of despair and tenderness', knowing that a child labelled a bastard must be 'an object of the greatest compassion' (p. 83). Attacked by her mistress and thrown out, Jemima eventually turns to abortion. Because her story is told in the first person, Wollstonecraft is able to offer a rare glimpse of a woman's feelings as the movements of the child in her body cease. The fact that the child moves is particularly significant in the context of contemporary debates about abortion, which was not actually criminalised until 1803. Prior to this, abortion was not a statutory offence, but was considered a 'misdemeanour' in common law and then only if it was procured after the stage of quickening. As Angus McLaren points out, 'as the woman herself was the only one to know if she had quickened and as attempts at abortion after four months would be rare, the law was in effect a dead letter'.[40] None the less, ecclesiastical tradition held that the foetus became 'ensouled' at the time of quickening, and from this perspective (one which, as a profoundly religious woman, Wollstonecraft might well have wished to endorse), Jemima has committed murder:[41]

I hurried back to my hole, and, rage giving place to despair, sought for the potion that was to procure abortion, and swallowed it, with a wish that it might destroy me, at the same time that it stopped the sensations of new-born life, which I felt with indescribable emotion. My head turned round, my heart grew sick, and in the horrors of approaching dissolution, mental anguish was swallowed up. (p. 84)

Despite or because of her suffering, when she finds a protector, Jemima in turn causes a girl who is pregnant by him to be turned out of his house. The girl subsequently commits suicide. Jemima describes herself as having been reduced at this point to a feral state: 'I was famishing: wonder not that I became a wolf!' (p. 89).

By far the most influential discussion of illegitimacy among the poorer classes was William Hunter's essay on infanticide, published four years before *Maria* in 1794. The essay was written in defence of women who were, in Hunter's view, often falsely accused of infanticide. Rather like Woolf's *Three Guineas*, it is framed as an expanded response to a letter, here from a country magistrate seeking Hunter's advice in defending a girl accused of infanticide. As Thomas Laqueur has pointed out, Hunter advances his argument in two distinct ways.[42] On the one hand, he marshals detailed physiological and pathological information to support his argument for the difficulty of establishing whether or not a child has been stillborn. For example, he argues against the infallibility of the 'floating lung test', in which a dead infant's lungs are placed in water. If they float, the child is assumed to have taken a breath: Hunter points out that the lungs may also float because of the effects of putrefaction. On the other hand, he deploys scenarios which are in effect case histories. He imagines an unmarried girl with 'an unconquerable sense of shame', drawn into concealment and disavowal of her pregnancy. 'In proportion as she loses the hope either of having been mistaken with regard to pregnancy, of being relieved from her terrors by a fortunate miscarriage, she every day sees her danger nearer and nearer, and her mind more overwhelmed by terror and despair.'[43] Hunter argues that women in this situation waver between different schemes for concealing the birth, but often go into labour sooner than expected, when their distress deprives them of 'all judgement'. Then,

> they are delivered by themselves, wherever they happened to retire in their fright and confusion; sometimes dying in the agonies of childbirth, and sometimes being quite exhausted, they faint away, and become insensible of what is passing; and when they recover a little strength, find that the child, whether still-born or not, is completely lifeless. In such a case, is it to be expected, when it could answer no purpose, that a woman should divulge the secret?' (pp. 10–11)

As Laqueur argues, Hunter makes his appeal on humanitarian grounds, inviting the reader to sympathise affectively with a fellow creature.

Indeed, in these case histories Hunter deploys rhetorical strategies not unlike those Wollstonecraft uses. The language is highly emotive: the words 'shame', 'terrors', 'terror and despair', 'fright and confusion' 'agonies' cluster together. In the passage quoted above, Hunter also suggests an analogy between the woman giving birth in solitude and a hunted animal.

On the surface, this text seems very different from Hunter's *Anatomia Uteri Humani Gravidi*. In the essay, scientific argument and humane feeling threaten to collide and are just held together, in creative tension. However, something of the same tension can be traced in the obstetrical atlas, in which the 'dispassionate' dissection of the torsos of dead women is counterbalanced, even infused by, specifically humane feeling. Hunter went out of his way to defend the objectivity of the new method of engraving used in his atlas: he claimed that 'the art of engraving supplies us, upon many occasions, with what has been the great *desideratum* of the lovers of science, an universal language' (Preface). However, like photography, also initially viewed as a transparent medium, the technique of engraving carries particular cultural meanings and was associated in the later eighteenth century with the depiction of harmonious natural landscapes (landscape being a new form) and portraiture. The engraver Jan van Rymsdyk's use of the medium in the *Anatomia* conferred humanity and integrity on Hunter's dead subjects, so that the atlas, like the essay on infanticide, bears witness to a productive tension between scientific and humane discourses.

While Wollstonecraft and Hunter focus sympathetically on illegitimacy among the poor, Frances Sheridan, in *The Memoirs of Miss Sidney Bidulph* (1761), explores the disruptive effects of illegitimacy among the upper classes, particularly in relation to the exploitation of pregnancy for financial/inheritance purposes. Illegitimacy intrudes into the life of the eponymous hero on two occasions. First, Sidney is forced to break off her engagement to Orlando Faulkland when it emerges that a Miss Burchell is already pregnant with his child. Various plot complications ensure that the full truth of the situation is withheld from Sidney: it finally transpires that Faulkland had only one encounter with Miss Burchell and that it was she who seduced him. None the less, even had she known the full facts, Sidney would still have renounced Faulkland and urged him to marry Miss Burchell, for she considers it his duty to take legal responsibility for a woman in a vulnerable position. She persists in this view even after her husband's death leads Faulkland to renew his addresses to her. She

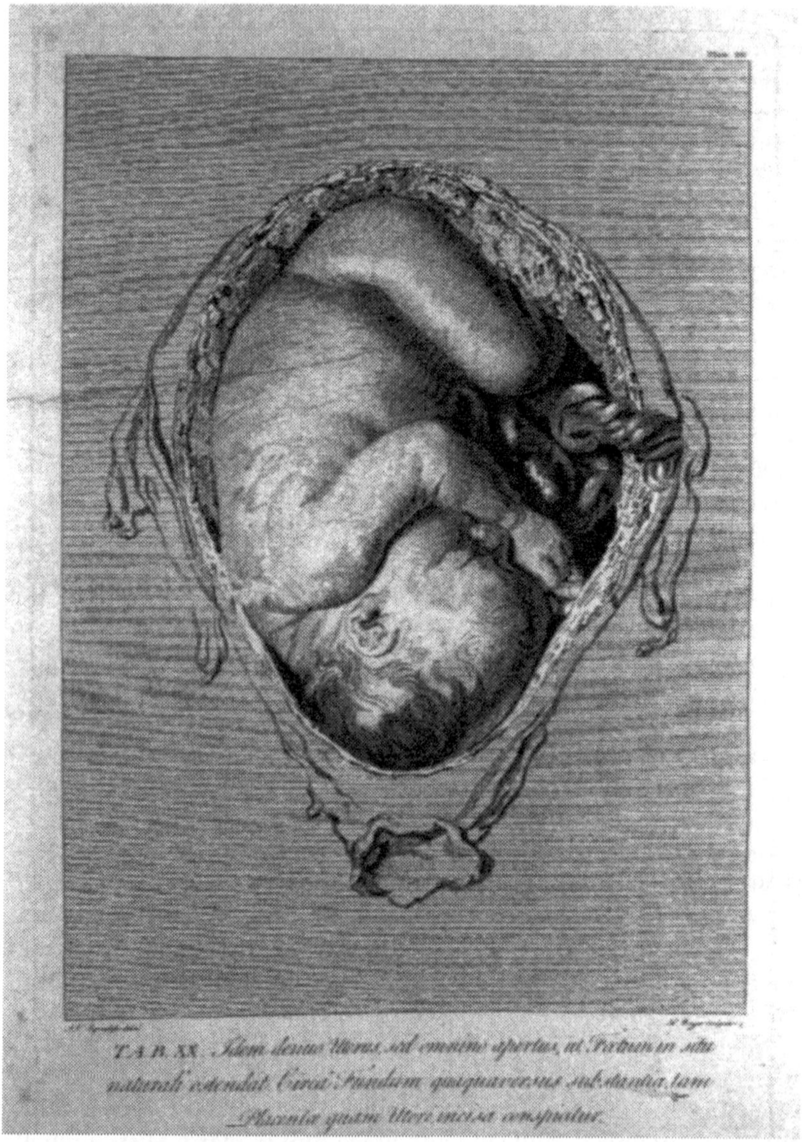

Figure 3   William Hunter, *The Anatomy of the Human Gravid Uterus*, 1774, Plate XX. Wellcome Library, London.

reflects on this occasion that 'there is nothing now to prevent me from warmly interfering for Miss Burchell. Charming young woman, how is she to be pitied! The tedious years of suspence, of almost hopeless love, that she has passed, deserve a recompence; and her little boy, my mother tells me, is a lovely creature.'[44] Miss Burchell turns out, however, to be a 'female rake', who has used her pregnancy to work on both Faulkner and Sidney Bidulph for financial gain. After her marriage to Faulkner she returns to a life of debauchery, and eventually dies 'unpitied and unlamented'. The lack of pity, endorsed through the narrative perspective, seems to have a good deal to do with the fact that Miss Burchell is represented as an upstart member of the expanding middle class, seeking to use reproduction as a form of production, a means of upward social mobility.

Illegitimacy intrudes into the narrative for a second time during Sidney's marriage to Mr Arnold. He expects to inherit his childless elder brother's estate, but the brother's widow has recourse to a manoeuvre which was then legally possible. Four months after her husband's death the widow finds she is pregnant and claims that this is the child of her dead husband. She and her husband were known to have lived apart, but a story of a reconciliation is cooked up, with a supporting witness who is probably the real father of the child. A protracted lawsuit follows which Mr Arnold is confident of winning, but the judgment goes against him and he and Sidney are reduced to near penury. As in the case of Miss Burchell, the widow is presented as a middle-class interloper, reflecting contemporary fears about the expanding middle class. Such cases produced frequent territorial struggles between doctors and lawyers, in which doctors were on weak ground because they were unable to rule with certainty on the possible duration of pregnancy, which was often the critical issue. As Montgomery emphasised, 'the purity of virtue, the honour and peace of domestic life, legitimacy, and the succession to rank, titles, and property, not infrequently depend solely for their invalidation or establishment on the settlement of this question' (p. 251). However, he had to admit that doctors could not pronounce with any finality. The law itself was not exact, assuming that pregnancy lasted nine calendar months or forty weeks, periods which were not identical. Moreover, authorities such as Hamilton and Denman had taken the view that, on occasion, gestation could be protracted for weeks beyond the normal term. Under such uncertain circumstances, strategies like those adopted by the widow had a considerable chance of success, and Montgomery gives several examples of such 'feigning'.

It was not only questions of pre- and post-maturity which rendered the concept of legitimacy unstable in this period: the legality of a marriage could be called in question. It could be a belated marriage, designed to confer a legitimacy which might be contested. This happens in *The Memoirs of Miss Sidney Bidulph*, when, after all Sidney's efforts on behalf of Miss Burchell and Faulkner's child, the illegitimacy of the child is 'proved' and Faulkner's estate is claimed by his family. Complications could also ensue if the marriage were between people of different faiths. In the case of the writer Fanny Burney and her husband Alexandre d'Arblay, for example, both Protestant and Catholic marriage services took place, to ensure that there could be no legal difficulties for any subsequent children. Charlotte Smith's daughter Augusta, like Burney, married a French revolutionary exile, and Smith had great difficulty in ensuring that both Protestant and Catholic ceremonies took place (an episcopal dispensation was necessary to secure this). This issue makes its way into her novel *Montalbert* (1795), in which the heroine, Rosalie, is drawn into a marriage of uncertain legal status. She is persuaded to marry in secret in a Catholic but not a Protestant ceremony, and it is never clear to her how binding this ceremony has been.[45] *Montalbert* explores the effects of illegitimacy across two generations: shortly after her marriage, Rosalie discovers that the woman she has always known as her mother's friend, and for whom she is named, is in fact her mother. The elder Rosalie's story demonstrates the greater opportunities available to the wealthy for concealing illegitimacy and avoiding disgrace. She knows that her father would never allow her to marry her lover, who is *déclassé*: in this sense her child is a literal embodiment of the transgression of class boundaries. However, in her privileged position she is able to deliver her child in secret and pass it off as another woman's: the cost is a loveless marriage.

Preformationism, epigenesis and *Frankenstein*

It has been pointed out that, despite the development of obstetrics in this period, many of the clinical aspects of pregnancy were little understood. There was little knowledge of the causes of foetal death, of miscarriage or of deformity at birth. However, the understanding of very early life (embryology) was changing rapidly and it was a subject which was fiercely debated. In the seventeenth century the invention of the microscope had enabled close study of the ovum and spermatozoon, and while scientists such as the Dutch naturalist

Jan Swammerdam had claimed to see complete miniature organisms in the ovum, others claimed that such organisms could be found in the sperm. Either way, it was believed that, at conception, the new individual was completely developed or 'preformed', and that during gestation it simply increased in size. In its most extreme variant, the doctrine of preformationism held that every human being was already formed in the first human creature. In the eighteenth century, however, the alternative theory of epigenesis was proposed, that is, that the various organs of the body are not all present at conception, but appear gradually during the formation of the foetus. Preformationism, with its deterministic religious overtones, was attractive to those of a conservative temperament such as Denman, who deployed the ingenious concept of 'unfolding' in an attempt to reconcile preformationism with what was then known of early embryonic development:

> It has been thought that some of the parts of the *foetus* were formed before the rest, and much labour hath been bestowed in ascertaining the order of their formation. But, as the skin of the smallest *embryo* which can be examined is perfect, it may be presumed that what has been called addition or coaptation of parts, is, in fact, nothing more than the expansion or unfolding of parts already formed. (p. 204)

Denman's intervention draws attention to an aspect of the problem, which we might now cast in terms of genetic rather than divine determination. To what extent is a developmental blueprint laid down at the moment of conception? How far do genes determine development, and what is the role of the environment, intra-uterine as well as postnatal?

Hunter's work seemed to contradict Denman's views. The last plate of the *Anatomia Uteri Humani Gravidi* (Plate 34) depicts conceptions at three, four and five weeks, and Hunter's gloss on the five-week embryo reads: 'The head of the *foetus* was longer than the trunk: the arms and legs had shot out but a little way: the abdominal *viscera* were not covered; the darker part of these was the red liver: there being no navel-string, the *foetus* was attached at its *abdomen* to the inside of the *amnion* and of the *chorion*, which were contiguous at that place.' Hunter's descriptions (and visual depictions) of partially formed organs may have influenced Erasmus Darwin, who was one of the most energetic exponents of the epigenetic view. In *Zoonomia*, Darwin scoffed at the 'ingenious philosophers' who supposed that all human progeny could have been contained in the first human being, for

> as these included embryons are supposed each of them to consist of the various and complicate part of animal bodies: they must possess a much greater degree of minuteness, than that which was ascribed to the devils that tempted St Anthony; of whom 20,000 were said to have been able to dance a saraband on the point of the finest needle. (Vol. 2, p. 490)

He went on to propound his theory of growth *in utero* via the 'apposition of parts', arguing that the child developed not through the extension of an already existent form, but through an accretive process which, crucially, involved some degree of interaction with the uterine environment:

> With every new change, therefore, of organic form, or addition of organic parts, I suppose a new kind of irritability or of sensibility to be produced; such varieties of irritability or of sensibility exist in our adult state in the glands; every one of which is furnished with an irritability, or a taste, or appetency, and a consequent mode of action peculiar to itself.
>
> In this manner I conceive the vessels of the jaws to produce those of the teeth, those of the fingers to produce the nails, those of the skin to produce the hair...These changes I conceive to be formed not by elongation or distention of primeval stamina, but by apposition of parts; as the mature crab-fish, when deprived of a limb, in a certain space of time has power to regenerate it. (Vol. 2, pp. 493–4)

Darwin emphasised the fact that the foetus could 'select' from the nutritive particles provided by the mother, thus construing the foetus as an active participant in gestation. However, by the same token, its development could be compromised by an inadequate maternal environment: it could 'be affected by the deficiency of the quantity of nutrition supplied by the mother, or by the degree of oxygenation supplied to its placenta by the maternal blood' (Vol. 2, p. 527).

Darwin's theory of generation was prescient and unusual in its emphasis on the potentially adverse effects the intra-uterine environment could have on foetal development. His work was known to both Percy and Mary Shelley, who refer to his poem *The Botanic Garden* as the source of conversations about the origin of life. He is also referred to in Percy Shelley's Preface to the 1818 edition of *Frankenstein* (written as from the author) and Mary Shelley's Preface to the revised 1831 edition. It was Ellen Moers who first argued that *Frankenstein* should be read as 'a birth myth' and since then there have been numerous readings of the creation of Frankenstein's monster in relation to real or imagined pregnancy. While Moers linked the text's theme with the biographical context of Mary Shelley's 'failed' pregnancies, later critics, such as Mary Jacobus and Barbara Johnson, have focused on Shelley's elision of the female body in the text. Alan Bewell has argued, however, that *Frankenstein* offers a meditation on the cultural linking of monstrosity and birth and 'an ambiguously female-based theory of creation in the Romantic discourse on the imagination', based on the notion of the creative power of the pregnant woman's imagination.[46] I would suggest that rather than exploring the creative power of the pregnant woman's imagination, *Frankenstein* considers the potentially destructive power of an inadequate uterine environment. Frankenstein works to create his 'child' by methods which echo Darwin's description of gestation taking place through the 'apposition of parts', and the whole process of construction resembles the physiologically-based descriptions of the epigenesists, whereby the child develops through 'successive accretions'. However, as Darwin points out, this process is not predetermined, but depends on a delicate balance of factors: the mother must provide the appropriate environment for the foetus. It is this that Frankenstein so signally fails to do, as he creates an artificial womb without light, while he himself works without nourishment, in an 'emaciated' state:

> In a solitary chamber, or rather cell, at the top of the house, and separated from all the other apartments by a gallery and staircase, I kept my workshop of filthy creation: my eyeballs were starting from their sockets in attending to the details of my employment. The dissecting room and the slaughter-house furnished many of my materials ...[47]

Small wonder that when the monster is 'born' it has the waxy appearance and 'dull yellow eye' of a sickly, undernourished baby. The landscape in which Frankenstein 'labours' at his second creation, a mate for the monster, is similarly marked by darkness and paucity of nourishment. It is a bare island on which '[t]he soil was barren, scarcely affording pasture for a few miserable cows, and oatmeal for its inhabitants, which consisted of five persons, whose gaunt and scraggy limbs gave tokens of their miserable fare' (p. 158). If Frankenstein had allowed the female monster to be born, we can infer, her 'scraggy limbs' would also have offered tokens of her 'miserable fare'.

We might therefore want to propose an alternative to the conventional linking of the monstrosity of Shelley's text with the articulation and/or critique of male structures of desire. Mary Jacobus argues that the novel is structured round Victor's 'intense identification with an oedipal conflict ... at the expense of identification with women', and Elizabeth Bronfen suggests that Frankenstein's monster 'competes with and repeals nature in an attempt to eliminate maternity entirely'.[48] Such positions assume that Shelley's main preoccupation is with male desire (and thus recast earlier readings of the text as a critique of male rationalism). However, one could turn this round and read the text in terms of female desire and its corollary, female fear. This would radically shift our reading of the terror which runs through the text and which is most vividly expressed in Victor's celebrated dream:

> I thought I saw Elizabeth, in the bloom of health, walking in the streets of Ingolstadt. Delighted and surprised, I embraced her, but as I imprinted the first kiss on her lips, they became livid with the hue of death; her features appeared to change, and I thought that I held the corpse of my dead mother in my arms; a shroud enveloped her form, and I saw the grave-worms crawling in the folds of flannel. (p. 57)

Rather than reading this in terms of male desire/fear of the maternal, we might do so in terms of female desire/fear. Specifically, we might read it in terms of fear of maternal failure, fear of being the bearer of death while desiring to give life. The worms within the shroud might thus figure harmful forces within the generative female body, more terrible than grave-worms because feeding on life. The deadly embrace with the mother might represent not a desire to eliminate the maternal but fear of standing in the place of the mother. To occupy this place is to risk not only one's own death, but that of the child one carries. Mary Wollstonecraft underlined this when she wrote of her fear that her emotional state in pregnancy would lead to her 'tormenting, or perhaps killing, a poor little animal, about whom I am grown anxious and tender'.[49] Although Shelley draws on epigenetic theory rather than the earlier notion of maternal impressions, she similarly explores in her novel the fear of 'tormenting, or perhaps killing' the child *in utero*.

2
Moral Physiology

Woman's nature

The early nineteenth century saw the emergence of a new genre, the medico-social text, which established relationships between and explored the imbrication of medical knowledge and social issues. In the field of reproduction, such texts typically considered the relationship between woman's physiology and her 'nature', and between the female (physical) economy and wider social structures. Such texts thus had a range far beyond that of the treatise on midwifery or advice book, claiming expertise and authority on social and philosophical as well as medical questions. They derived from a variety of political perspectives (often appearing in conjunctions surprising to the modern reader), but for the purposes of discussion they can be separated into two broad categories. The first is that of texts written by progressive reformers who were influenced by post-revolutionary radical politics. In Britain in this period progressive thought was closely linked with utopian movements such as Carlilean republicanism and Owenism. These movements, in turn, were founded on a critique of all aspects of social organisation, including marriage and family structure. Robert Owen, for example, argued flamboyantly that

> the present marriages of the world, under the system of moral evil in which they have been devised and are now contracted, are the sole cause of all the prostitution, of all its incalculable grievous evils, and of more than one half of all the vilest and most degrading crimes known to society.[1]

In some radical circles, women's rights were debated and considered in relation not only to civic and legal issues, but also to such questions as domestic violence and, crucially, women's control over their fertility. In opening up the question of birth control such thinkers addressed an issue which the previous generation (including Godwin and Wollstonecraft) had been unable or unwilling to discuss in public. It remained a particularly sensitive issue, because the dissemination of information about family limitation could be linked with a Malthusian agenda of controlling the numbers of the labouring poor. For this reason, those writers who promoted birth control went out of their way to emphasise the benefits it would bring to the poor in terms of improved health and opportunities for financial advancement. It was also implied that the aristocracy had practised birth control for generations, but had deliberately sought to withhold this advantage from the poorer classes. Richard Carlile argued that contraception was the only remedy for 'the unemployed, ill-employed, and badly paid, surplus population', and that it had long been known to the aristocracy, 'who are always in search of benefits which they can peculiarly hold, and be distinct from the body of the labouring people'.[2]

Carlile was a republican who began to express his radical views about women's political and sexual position during the years 1819–25, when he was imprisoned in Newgate for publishing 'blasphemous material' (translations of the works of Tom Paine). In 1828 he published a short pamphlet on contraception, *Every Woman's Book; or, What is Love?* One of the main strands of his argument here was that the free expression of sexual desire was necessary for the health of both men and women; in his words, 'Love must be gratified, or its victim wastes and dies.' Carlile attempted to ground this claim in contemporary physiological knowledge, although the evidence he offered was, to say the least, anecdotal:

> One of our principal London physicians, in conversation on female disorder, observed to a lady, that *in nine cases out of ten of sickness, and in five cases out of six of death from consumption, among young women, the proximate cause was the want of sexual commerce.* He added, *the present state of society will not admit of my saying this publicly; but such is the fact, and it would be well if it were more generally known.* (p. 21; Carlile's emphasis)

As this passage suggests, while Carlile stressed his belief in equality, *Every Woman's Book* also reveals potential points of fracture and conflicts of interest between the sexes. On occasion it reads like a manifesto for free love and, as Barbara Taylor has pointed out, in the

1820s as in the 1960s arguments for the unfettered indulgence of the 'passion of love' could pose a serious threat to women's interests.[3] It is also significant that Carlile focuses on equality of passions and desires: in the main, his advocacy of birth control is located in a discourse emphasising sexual rather than social freedoms. None the less, in common with Francis Place's 1822 *Illustrations and Proofs of the Principle of Population*, *Every Woman's Book* made available information about the withdrawal method and the French letter (*baudruche*), and Carlile drew on all his propagandist skills in an attempt to persuade women of the convenience of the sponge, his favoured method of contraception:

> The important discovery is, that if, before sexual intercourse, the female introduces into her vagina a piece of sponge as large as can be pleasantly introduced, having previously attached a bobbin or bit of narrow riband to withdraw it, it will be found a preventive to conception ...
>
> The practice is common with the females of the more refined parts of the continent of Europe, and with those of the Aristocracy of England. An English Duchess was lately instanced to the writer, who never goes out to a dinner without being prepared with the sponge. French and Italian women wear them fastened to their waists, and always have them at hand. (pp. 38–9)

Robert Dale Owen's *Moral Physiology; or, a Brief and Plain Treatise on the Population Question*, published two years later, has a very different emphasis. Owen defines his subject as 'strictly physiological, although connected, like many other physiological subjects, with political economy, morals, and social science'.[4] Like Carlile, he emphasises the value of sexual pleasure for both sexes. Sexual abstinence, he argues, is damaging, causing 'peevishness and melancholy', whereas the exercise of the reproductive instinct has an influence which is 'moral, humanizing, polishing, beneficent' (p. 11). However, Owen locates such pleasure in the context of marriage, and his advocacy of birth control is in the interests of greater happiness and equity within marriage. *Moral Physiology* is, moreover, one of the first texts to make the connection between women's oppression and continual maternity. Owen analyses the asymmetrical relationship of men and woman to reproduction, and asks:

> in how many instances does the hard-working father, and more especially the mother of a poor family, remain slaves throughout

their lives, tugging at the oar of incessant labour, toiling to live, and living only to die ... How often is the health of the mother – giving birth, every year, perchance, to an infant – happy, if it be not twins! – and compelled to toil on, even at those times when nature imperiously calls for some relief from daily drudgery – how often is the mother's comfort, health, nay, her life, thus sacrificed!' (p. 20)

He goes on to consider the adverse effects of repeated childbearing not just on women's health, but on their freedom and autonomy, questioning whether, for example, 'the whole life of an intellectual, cultivated woman, should be spent in bearing a family of twelve or fifteen children' (p. 24).

Although Owen, like Carlile, advocated the use of contraception as a means of improving the condition of the poor, his primary interest was in the reform of sexual relations. Living in the New Harmony community founded by his father, Robert Owen, in America, he edited the radical feminist paper the *Free Enquirer* between 1828 and 1832, and with his wife Mary Robinson campaigned for reform of women's legal position in Indiana. In *Moral Physiology* he tackled not just the question of inequity within marriage but also outside it, mounting a forthright attack on the sexual double standard, with particular reference to pregnancy. He noted that if an unmarried woman became pregnant, though her offence was 'but an error of judgement or a weakness of the heart', the consequence was the same as if 'her imprudence were indeed a crime of the blackest dye'. He continued:

> And, let me ask, what is it gives to the arts of seduction their sting, and stamps to the world its victim? Why is it, that the man goes free and enters society again, almost courted and applauded, while the women is a mark for the finger of reproach, and a butt for the tongue of scandal? *Is it not chiefly because she bears about her the mark of what is called her disgrace? She becomes a mother*; and society has something tangible against which to direct its anathemas. Nine-tenths, at least, of the misery and ruin which are caused by seduction, even in the present state of public opinion, result from cases of pregnancy. (pp. 27–8; emphasis added)

However, although Owen focuses firmly on the plight of the unmarried mother (she and her child are described as 'a dove in the falcon's claws' of society), he finds himself unable to recommend either the sponge or the baudruche (which was indeed extremely expensive) as methods of contraception. Coitus interruptus is the only method he finds agreeable and convenient; it is also, as he acknowledges, only at the disposal of the man. Thus his radical project founders to the extent that the control of reproduction remains in the hands of men.

The radicalism of *Moral Physiology* is also qualified or tempered by a strand of elitism which is evident in Owen's interest in the 'intellectual, cultivated woman' noted above. This tendency finds fuller expression in a proto-eugenic argument which develops out of his consideration of women who suffer repeated stillbirths. He goes on to argue that there are some people who should never become parents, because if they do they will transmit to their children 'grievous hereditary diseases; perhaps that worst of diseases, insanity'. To do so is 'an immorality'. However, if such people refrained from becoming parents, the health of the race would benefit enormously: 'Who can estimate the beneficial effects which rational, moral restraint may thus have on the physical improvement of our race, throughout future ages!' (p. 21). Strikingly, Owen uses the metaphor of 'poisoned fruit' to describe children born with a hereditary disease. This was deployed quite frequently in late nineteenth-century eugenic discourse, but, as has been argued in chapter 1, eugenic thought has a longer pre-history than is often appreciated.

Carlile and Owen were not medically trained, but drew on medico-scientific discourse to support their arguments for 'moral [ethical] physiology'. In contrast, Emma Martin, an Owenite reformer, had trained as a midwife and used her training to inform and support her arguments for women's control over their own bodies. Martin was a utilitarian and rationalist who published in the mid-century a series of pamphlets attacking religion. Among other things, she offered a sophisticated feminist critique of biblical ideology, attacking the mixture of prurience and misogyny which informed the representation of women in many biblical texts. She argued that the influence of Christianity in Victorian culture was damaging to women, purveying false notions about their sexuality. In her pamphlet *The Bible No Revelation, or the Inadequacy of Language to convey A Message from God to Man*, she argued that girls should be given 'scientific information' about their bodies:

> I am far from supposing that ignorance is one of virtue's safe-guards, and would have scientific information given to all. Especially to the future mothers of our race, would I have the 'Knowledge of themselves,' the laws of their own nature, the accidents and requirements of themselves and their probable offspring, imparted. ...

I would rather give my daughters a set of physiological and obstetric books for their perusal, than allow them to read the Levitical law, or the stories of the two Tamars, of Bathsheba, Lot, and others, and I know that while the one will give information which may be serviceable, and which can never generate premature passion, the other is calculated to confound the distinctions of right and wrong.[5]

Apart from this plea for sex education, Martin offers a robust challenge to the use of religion to support views of women's reproductive function as unmentionable and/or unclean. The reference in the passage quoted above to Leviticus, which advocates the purification of women after pregnancy and childbirth, is especially pointed (Leviticus 12).

Those writers who offered a more conservative perspective on women and reproduction were in the main medically qualified, though this does not mean that their views were representative of the profession as a whole.[6] In the mid-century, writers such as William Acton and William Carpenter became extremely well known, and their views on such issues as women's intellectual inferiority and sexual passivity were taken up by other commentators in the emerging specialisms of psychology and social science. However, as historians have emphasised, the fact that these ideas were widely circulated must not be taken as an indication that women's consciousness or behaviour was significantly modified by them. Rather, the writings of Acton, Carpenter and others might be read as expressive of male anxieties in response to women's increasing engagement in public life and debate in this period. In the early to mid-nineteenth century, women could and did participate in public life through involvement in radical politics as well as through widespread community and philanthropic endeavours. In the same period, writers such as Owen and Emma Martin offered provocative readings of women's intellectual abilities *and* sexual nature. It is in such a context that we must consider works such as John Power's influential *Essays on the Female Economy*, published in 1821. By 'female economy', Power means female physiology, and from this point of view the most significant contribution of his book is its argument for the (previously unrecognised) connection between ovulation and menstruation. More influential, however, was his treatment of menstruation as a 'natural' process. He argued that if women were living 'in a state of nature', menstruation would be unknown, for between the ages of fifteen and forty-five, 'one nine months would be employed in producing, and the next nine months in nourishing, her child, so that no time would be left for its occurrence'.[7] Moscucci interprets this in terms of the advocacy of continuous (natural) reproduction for women, but this is not Power's position.[8] Instead, he develops the paradoxical concept of a 'second nature' which prevents women from exerting their natural powers of reproduction. He argues that the hymen, which is peculiar to the human female,

> has, without doubt, some relation to her moral state, and may be considered as an evidence that the wise Creator intended to place restraints on the sexual passions of the human race, and their consequences, and is a fine illustration of the difference of its relations with its beneficent author, from those of the inferior animals. Our moral and religious duties are not infrequently at variance with the dictates of nature; and it is to this seeming contradiction that the present paradox must be referred. (pp. 28–9)

It is the human female who exercises 'natural' restraint and whose sexual passivity curbs human passions. None the less, women, though passive, must maintain their bodies as efficient reproductive machines and to this end must not engage in too much intellectual work. Here Power ties together concerns about women's education and about differential breeding (as later nineteenth-century writers were to do). He warns of the ill-effects of modern education on the health of 'young ladies', in particular through their 'confinement to sedentary and monotonous occupation'. Young women need freedom of bodily exertion, for '[t]he acquisitions of intellectual power, or of individual accomplishment ... are often dearly purchased by the sacrifice of health, and a proportionate debility of bodily power; and hence obstructed menstruation is so prevalent amongst the higher classes of society' (p. 61).

Commentators like Alexander Walker continued the double (and somewhat contradictory) project of asserting woman's sexual passivity while at the same time identifying her almost exclusively with the reproductive function. In *Woman, Physiologically Considered as to Mind, Morals, Marriage, Matrimonial Slavery, Infidelity and Divorce* (1839), he argued that woman's mental activity was instinctive rather than rational because of her specialised function: 'It is so evident as scarcely to require mention, that love, impregnation, gestation, parturition, lactation, and nursing, have little or nothing to do with reason, and are almost entirely instinctive.' He goes on to claim that women's morals derive from her reproductive role, which also modifies her intellect:

> it will be seen ... that [woman's] relations to every thing around her, and consequently her morals ...·are all either absolutely created, or powerfully modified, by her instinctive vital system ... It will, moreover, appear that the fundamental and essential character of the mental and locomotive systems of woman are, owing to their slighter development, utterly incapable of rising above this instinctive influence of her vital system.[9]

He concludes, robustly, that 'Hence, when Mrs Wolstonecraft [*sic*] says, "I may be allowed to infer that reason is absolutely necessary to enable a woman to perform any duty properly," she infers nonsense' (pp. 24–5). For Walker, rational activity is not only unnecessary for woman's 'function' but detrimental to it.

Walker's text also demonstrates the link between the idea of maternal impressions and of the insanity of pregnancy. He notes women's susceptible imagination, which he ascribes to 'the peculiar and distinctive influence of the matrix', and goes on to claim that such is the power of this faculty that even 'those who possess most reason and strength of mind, frequently give way under a certain state of the body, as at the approach of the catamenia, or during the first months of pregnancy', and become mentally deranged (p. 30). Having painted this picture of women as creatures whose mental and moral faculties are subordinate to their reproductive system, he goes on to debar them from any part in government or legislation on *practical* grounds. For Walker, pregnancy represents an insuperable problem: women, if admitted to Parliament, would be affected by the symptoms and diseases of gestation, and even, perhaps, by premature parturition. Were a tendency to the latter 'to spread rapidly among the congregated female senators, as it does sometimes among the females of inferior animals, what a scene would ensue! A few midwives, to be sure, might be added to the officers of the house. Thus a man might have the glory, not merely of having died, like Lord Chatham, in the senate, but of having been born there!' (p. 69).

Such recourse to an analogy between women and animals is frequent in texts on women's nature, physiology or economy; as Jill Matus has pointed out, a focus on the form and function of such analogies 'highlights the ideological dimension involved in interpreting plant and animal reproductive behaviour in relation to that of human beings' – although it is important to recognise that it was also the case that much physiological knowledge could then, as now, only be derived from experimental work on non-human subjects.[10] The analogy is certainly used in varied ways – while Walker yokes together women and 'the inferior animals', Power was concerned to establish a categorical distinction between morally responsible human beings (women being the pre-eminent bearers of sexual morality) and 'the inferior animals'. Other commentators such as William Acton deployed the comparison in a relatively neutral fashion. Acton's well-known tract on *The Functions and Disorders of the Reproductive Organs* (1857), which went into many editions, was primarily concerned with the sexual health of men and the need to 'husband' men's reproductive resources. Not surprisingly in view of this concern, Acton was also one of the commentators who emphasised the sexual passivity of women. He argued that 'the majority of women (happily for society) are not very much troubled with sexual feeling of any kind' and claimed too that '[i]f the married female conceives every second year, we usually notice that during the nine months following conception she experiences no great sexual excitement. The consequence is that sexual desire in the male is somewhat diminished, and the act of coition takes place but rarely.'[11] Acton goes on to note that, in this respect, women differ very little from 'the females among animals', writing that 'certainly, during the months of gestation this holds good. I have known instances where the female has during gestation evinced positive loathing for any marital familiarity whatever. In some exceptional cases, indeed, feeling has been sacrificed to duty, and the wife has endured, with all the self-martyrdom of womanhood, what was almost worse than death' (p. 213). Acton represents woman as passive, especially during pregnancy, because that is *the* state in which her purity needs to be demonstrated, not least to the anxious male. For as contemporary writers were beginning to suggest, women must maintain complete moral as well as physical hygiene if they were to reproduce satisfactorily. As Thomas Laycock put it,

When a woman has lost her modesty, her fitness to procreate off-spring of high moral excellence is probably lost too. Certainly she is no longer either a suitable companion or a solace for her husband, or a fit teacher and trainer for her children. To a man of high moral purity an immodest woman, however attractive corporeally and sensually, is an object of repugnance.[12]

The ideological project of such medico-social texts is to construct woman as a passionless reproductive being, for whom too much mental activity is contraindicated as it may jeopardise reproductive success. Indulgence in intellectual pursuits among women was, paradoxically, considered to be extremely common *and* unnatural, requiring strong external and internal controls. There were some commentators who dissented from the view of woman as passionless: W. Tyler Smith, for example, in his *Manual of Obstetrics: Theoretical and Practical* noted that

> The female is considered 'passive,' both by Prof. Muller and Dr. Carpenter, during coitus, but this is evidently a mistake. The sexual 'paroxysm' in the female was fully recognised by John Hunter, and is as distinct as that of the male. It begins in the clitoris, and ends in an orgasm or paroxysm of sensation ... It should be observed, however, that the orgasm is not at all necessary to conception.[13]

However, the ascription of sexual appetite to women did not lead to their being seen as active sexual agents, but was interpreted instead in terms of their subjection to the procreative instinct.

The insanity of pregnancy

The mental and emotional powers which such commentators wished to dissociate from pregnancy returned with a vengeance, however, in the form of the disease category and symptoms of the 'insanity of pregnancy'. This is a phenomenon which has received surprisingly little attention from historians of medicine and culture. In order to understand it, some assumptions about the construction of disease categories need to be disentangled. In the past, following Michel Foucault, many historians have emphasised the power of medical institutions and taxonomies to regulate and normalise human behaviour among both sexes. It has also been argued by feminist historians that disease categories, particularly in relation to mental illness, have reflected and enforced male physicians' preconceptions about normal, neurotic or insane female behaviour.[14] The strength of such approaches lies in their sensitivity to the cultural components of disease and their awareness of the power of the medical establishment to create categories of disease, particularly in relation to mental illness: their weakness lies in a neglect of the input of the patient. Other historians have focused on the role of the patient in the construction of illness and have interpreted some illnesses (such as anorexia) as forms of cultural protest.[15] This has the advantage of situating disease in a specific social and cultural context, but risks overemphasis on disease as heroic resistance. In the case of the insanity of pregnancy, it is more accurate to see the illness as one that was jointly constructed by the medical profession and female patients, but that was differently inflected for these two groups. In this respect, the distinction Nancy Theriot makes between illness and disease is useful.[16] Theriot suggests that illness can be defined as a behaviour pattern involving mental and physical symptoms, whereas disease is the definition given by physicians to the illness symptoms. In considering discussions of the insanity of pregnancy in medical texts, it is often helpful to distinguish between the reported symptoms (often given in the form of narrative case histories) and the disease classification.

The idea that pregnancy could be associated with extreme despondency and even mental derangement first began to be canvassed in obstetric texts of the 1820s and 1830s. Douglas Fox, in *Signs, Disorders and Management of Pregnancy ...Written Expressly for the Use of Females*, noted that on the establishment of pregnancy 'innumerable sympathies arise throughout the system, producing not only extraordinary bodily sensations, as pains in the head, in the teeth, in the extremities, and in other parts, but often giving rise to the most singular mental irritations manifested by anxiety and despondency'.[17] The terms he uses ('sympathies', 'irritations') point to the connection between maternal impressions and the insanity of pregnancy. However, where maternal impressions were linked with susceptibility to emotion in a fairly broad sense, the idea of the insanity of pregnancy developed out of specific accounts of despondency. Fox noted, for example, that women 'possessing the most lively dispositions, as well as others, sometimes become extremely depressed and apprehensive during pregnancy, and view every object through a gloomy medium ... and life, which had previously been a state of enjoyment, is rendered an insupportable burden' (p. 58). W.F. Montgomery similarly wrote that in pregnancy, 'the irritation of the nervous system is in some most obviously perceived in the change induced in the moral temperament, rendering the individual depressed and despondent'. In extreme cases, 'the woman is constantly under the influence of a settled and gloomy anticipation of evil, sometimes accompanied with that sort of apathetic indifference which makes her careless of every object that ought naturally to awaken an interest in her feelings'.[18]

In the same period, in accordance with the ever-increasing special-isation of the medical profession, books on insanity were being published by doctors who took a special interest in the treatment of madness. The period between 1820 and 1860 was one of relative benevolence in the treatment of the insane. It was the age of the asylum (a term deliberately chosen to denote care rather than the carceral), and the doctrine of the 'moral management' of certain forms of insanity. While it was widely believed that madness had an organic basis (and many attempts were made to prove this), it was also accepted that insanity could be triggered by social and psycho-logical factors. Such cases were generally grouped under the rubric of 'moral insanity', a term introduced by James Pritchard in 1835 and defined in terms of 'a morbid perversion of the natural feelings, affections, inclinations, temper, habits, moral dispositions, and natural impulses, without any remarkable disorder or defect of the intellect'. Following J.E.D. Esquirol, whose work on insanity was carried out in the Salpêtrière, the asylum in which Freud was to 'discover' hysteria in 1895, Pritchard included the insanity of pregnancy in this category, writing that:

> Symptoms of insanity occasionally display themselves during preg-nancy, and under circumstances which indicate that they are dependent on that state ... M. Esquirol mentions the instance of a young woman of very sensitive habit who had attacks of madness on two occasions, each of which lasted fifteen days, having commenced immediately after conception.[19]

George Man Burrows, on the other hand, in his *Commentaries on the Causes, Forms, Symptoms, and Treatment, Moral and Medical, of Insanity*, placed mental illness in pregnancy in the category of 'genuine insan-ity', emphasising too the hereditary (and hence organic) causes of such insanity:

> Gestation itself is a source of excitation in most women, and some-times provokes mental derangement, and more especially in those with an hereditary predisposition. The accession of mental disturbance may be coincident with conception, and cease on quickening; or it may come on at any time during pregnancy, continue through it, and terminate with delivery, or persevere through all the circumstances consequent on parturition. Some are insane on every pregnancy or lying-in, others only occasionally.

Whenever mental disturbance occurs during pregnancy, it partakes oftener of an idiopathic character, either in the form of mania or melancholia, than of the delirium which succeeds parturition.[20]

Such differences in classification had implications for treatment. In cases where the physician took the view that mental disturbance in pregnancy had a primarily organic and/or hereditary cause, this was often associated with a diagnosis of mania, and the treatment was likely to involve some form of restraint. In his *Three Hundred Consultations in Midwifery*, Robert Lee thus gives an account of attending a patient who had been 'in a state of insanity' during pregnancy and whose near relation had destroyed himself in a fit of mania. During labour the patient became 'ungovernable'. Having ascertained that the child was dead, craniotomy was adopted to terminate both the labour and the mania. As noted in the Introduction, this was a painful and messy procedure. In another case, Lee describes the treatment adopted for a patient suffering from violent mania in the sixth month of pregnancy:

The question in this case was whether premature labour should be induced. The patient was in such a violent condition that it would not have been possible to have safely passed up the instrument into the uterus and perforated the membranes, if it had been considered necessary to do this. I recommended proper restraint, shaving the head, cold lotions, leeches to the temples, and giving cathartic medicine. The symptoms gradually diminished in intensity, and I believe the patient was safely delivered, and ultimately recovered perfectly.[21]

Such intrusive measures effectively constituted an assault on the pregnant woman, the aim, in accordance with theories of hereditary insanity, being social control as much as therapeutic intervention.

If, on the other hand, such disturbance were classified as moral insanity (more often associated with melancholia), the treatment would be 'moral management'. The assumption behind moral management was that if the mad were treated with kindness and placed in a calm and supportive environment, their symptoms would abate as their confidence and self-esteem returned. While such a prescription failed to comprehend (in both senses) the wilder shores of insanity, it was clearly an improvement on methods of mechanical restraint and showed sensitivity to the social contexts of insanity. In relation to the insanity of pregnancy, this was the approach most often adopted, and it brought the beginnings of an analysis of the reasons for women's misery in pregnancy. Dr J.B. Tuke (one of the family who had established a model asylum in the York Retreat in the early nineteenth century), published a key paper on the subject in 1865. He had studied types of puerperal insanity (pre- and postnatal, and in labour) and began his discussion of the insanity of pregnancy, startlingly, by emphasising the risk of suicide in such cases:

> In the insanity of pregnancy the symptoms are as a rule of a melancholic type ... In no form of insanity is the suicidal tendency so well marked: 13 patients, or nearly half, had either attempted or meditated suicide. In some the attempts were most determined, a loathing of life and intense desire to get rid of it being the actuating motives ... One patient, who was admitted after attempting suicide, and who made a rapid recovery, became insane during her next pregnancy; her friends hoped to be able to manage her at home; the result was she succeeded in poisoning herself.[22]

Tuke here made explicit what was implicit in earlier accounts of pregnant women's finding life 'an insupportable burden', and his account of the treatment offered in the Morningside Asylum points to some of the causes of insanity and/or suicidal impulses:

> The assurance of protection, the regularity, amusements, and employment alone to be found in an asylum, – above all, the freedom from domestic anxiety and the misapplied sympathy of relatives, – in a large majority of cases are productive of the best results. It is impossible for the class from which the large proportion of our patients is derived to obtain these advantages elsewhere. (p. 1016)

Pregnant women of all classes were subject to constant surveillance and control (under the guise of 'sympathy') from their families, and poorer women often experienced their pregnancies in extremely stressful domestic circumstances.

Tuke was aligned with the tradition of enlightened reform and moral management of the insane, which broadly held sway until the 1860s. However, by then the asylum system was coming under attack, partly for practical reasons, as it was thought that the sheer numbers of patients being admitted meant that the personal care advocated by the asylums' founders could no longer be provided. More crucial in its effects on the care of the insane, however, was the impact of Darwinian thought, nowhere more evident than in the life and work of Henry Maudsley, founder of the Maudsley Hospital and influential exponent of an early version of evolutionary psychiatry. Psychiatric Darwinists such as Maudsley took the view that evolution worked through the selection of the best mental as well as physical characteristics. Insanity was the result of an hereditary disposition to madness and represented a congenital inferiority, which would be passed on to future generations. Accordingly, the insane required not care and sustenance, but control, and should not be encouraged to breed. Such views migrated inevitably into the discussion of the insanity of pregnancy. Tuke himself had noted in his paper that such insanity was often linked with 'moral insanity ... dipsomania being the most common symptom', but Maudsley recast this in terms of hereditary moral perversion. In his first, and extremely influential, book *The Physiology and Pathology of Mind*, he wrote that 'in the insanity of pregnancy the symptoms are as a rule of a melancholic type; and in no other form of the disease [i.e. melancholia] is the suicidal tendency stronger. There is not uncommonly a considerable amount of moral perversion, so that the patient acts in a way which she would be heartily ashamed of if she were well.'[23] This perception was repeated in obstetric textbooks of the 1870s. William Leishman noted that the insanity of pregnancy was 'generally characterised by melancholia, or by moral perversion', and W.S. Playfair suggested that it was commonly associated with dipsomania and even kleptomania:

> Laycock mentions a disposition to 'kleptomania' as very characteristic of the disease. Casper relates a curious case where this occurred in a pregnant lady of rank, and the influence of pregnancy, in developing an irresistible tendency, was pleaded in a criminal trial in which one of her petty thefts had involved her.[24]

While melancholia continued to be listed as the most common symptom of the insanity of pregnancy, the incorporation of 'moral perversions' into the accepted group of symptoms was clearly linked with the rise of psychiatric Darwinism and posed a particular problem. While 'moral insanity' in pregnancy could be linked with social contexts (poverty and illegitimacy, most notably), hereditary insanity was considered to be inherent and unavoidable, and its manifestation in pregnancy could therefore be taken to suggest that the pregnant woman was 'unfit' to breed.

The most powerful representation of the insanity of pregnancy, and the most searching exploration of its symptoms and causes, occurs in one of the central texts of Victorian literature, *Wuthering Heights* (1847). Emily Brontë would have known of the disease from the Brontës' medical manuals, which included William Buchan's *Domestic Medicine* and Thomas Graham's *Modern Domestic Medicine*. Graham offers a particularly suggestive model of the illness, positing a combination of 'moral and physical causes' which can prey at a distance on 'the organs of generation' to produce madness or melancholy. He vividly invokes the repertoire of symptoms associated with the two different categories of insanity: madness involves 'an altered and peculiar appearance of the eyes, protruding and wild; rapid and successive change of features; unusual vigour and uncommon agitation of the whole muscular powers; insusceptibility to extremes of heat and cold', while the symptoms of melancholy, by contrast, can include 'great apathy; obstinate disposition to dwell upon some mournful topic; sleeplessness; pertinacious silence, and other symptoms of morbid intensity of thought'. Graham also suggests that 'madness very frequently terminates in the opposite form, or melancholy'.[25]

Catherine Linton's pregnancy is at the heart of *Wuthering Heights*, literally and figuratively, and represents the completion of the 'wounding' process begun on her first visit to Thrushcross Grange. In their classic reading of the novel, Sandra Gilbert and Susan Gubar argue that when Cathy is bitten at the Grange by the Linton's dog Skulker, with his phallic 'huge, purple tongue', she is 'catapulted into adult female sexuality'.[26] It would be more accurate to say that this is the beginning of a process whereby Cathy's body (and her body-ego) become alienated from her, as she is inducted into the structures of middle-class property and propriety. On her return to Wuthering Heights, she is described as having changed from 'a wild, hatless little savage' into a 'very dignified person, with brown ringlets falling from the cover of a feathered beaver, and a long cloth habit which she was obliged to hold up with both hands that she might sail in'.[27] She has transformed herself into an appropriate object for the wealthy Edgar Linton, and goes on to marry him despite her love for Heathcliff, who is 'more myself than I am'. Her first illness occurs before her marriage when Heathcliff runs off into the night, but this is an organic disease, a fever contracted after a night spent in wet clothes. Her second illness begins after a quarrel with Edgar and Heathcliff, when she is four and a half months pregnant. After Heathcliff's return to Wuthering Heights, he has visited her regularly despite her marriage, but Edgar eventually finds these visits unbearable and demands that she chooses between himself and Heathcliff, for '[i]t is impossible for you to be *my* friend, and *his* at the same time' (p. 156). Faced with this choice, Cathy's 'furious' answer is 'I require to be let alone!' in other words, she refuses to choose. She is, or feels she is, unable to do without the cultural (and economic) support provided by Linton, but nor can she continue without the 'self' represented by her double, Heathcliff. She alternates between rage and despair at Linton's ultimatum, dashing her head against the sofa, then stretching out in an attitude of death, and finally adopts the classic pose of the madwoman: 'she started up – her hair flying over her shoulders, her eyes flashing, the muscles of her neck and arms standing out preternaturally' (p. 157). She then locks herself in her room, to emerge in a state of 'feverish bewilderment'. Her illness is clearly mental rather than physical, and there are hints of a link with the irritability of pregnancy: Cathy's blood rushes 'into a hell of a tumult at a few words' and she is 'maddened' by injuries (p. 163).

This 'insanity' is compounded by a complex crisis of identity. When she emerges from her room, Cathy is unable to recognise herself in the mirror, seeing instead an alien, ghost-like presence:

> 'Don't *you* see that face?' she enquired, gazing earnestly at the mirror.
> And say what I could, I was incapable of making her comprehend it to be her own; so I rose and covered it with a shawl.
> 'It's behind there still!' she pursued, anxiously. 'And it stirred. Who is it? I hope it will not come out when you are gone! Oh! Nelly, the room is haunted! I'm afraid of being alone!' (p.161)

Twentieth-century psychoanalysts have argued that pregnancy creates a crisis of identity in terms of both inner and outer perceptions of the self. The body-ego is compromised, as the body no longer feels as though it occupies its 'own' space, and the ego-ideal represented by the mirror image is also threatened. As Lemoine-Luccioni explains in her idiosyncratic but suggestive study *The Dividing of Women or Woman's Lot* [*Partage des Femmes*]:

> Pregnancy is a narcissistic crisis ending in pseudo-delusion and depression ... because the ego-ideal, the specular image, is massively altered, putting to the test the she-narcissus who wants to remain the same, unchanging and outside of time (losing, what's more, the possibility of also 'stopping' time).[28]

The self created in the 'mirror stage' comes under pressure as the body visibly acts out process and generation, reminding the subject that she cannot 'stop' time, but must submit to bodily changes, which will end only with her death. To this extent, pregnancy also represents a move-ment to the place of the mother, a place which is outside, or prior to, identity, a shadow world. Lemoine-Luccioni describes the process in these terms: 'In place of the luminous double of the specular image, a shadow moves in, the obscure maternal double. The subject, then, allows the mirror to dull, to become leaden' (p. 33). This is, perhaps, the ghost Cathy sees in the mirror, both her mother's ghost and her own, as she falls back into a space before language, over-whelmed, as she says, by 'utter blackness' and with 'no command of tongue, or brain' (p. 162).

Cathy's pregnancy also, of course, commits her finally and irrevo-cably to her socio-reproductive role (Edgar has been hoping for an heir, Nelly Dean tells us, to secure his lands 'from a stranger's gripe'). It places her definitively as 'Mrs Linton, the lady of Thrushcross Grange, and the wife of a stranger', who wishes only to be a girl again 'half savage and hardy, and free' – not tamed, debili-tated and imprisoned. Her sense of imprisonment is most powerfully expressed in a reworking of Ophelia's mad scene, itself the *locus clas-sicus*, as Showalter and others have pointed out, of the representa-tion of female madness.[29] Her hair down (signifying sensuality and loss of self-control), Cathy shreds her pillow, scattering feathers over her room like snow, telling over their individual characteristics just as Ophelia tells over the qualities of herbs ('There's fennel for you, and columbines ...'):

> 'That's a turkey's,' she murmured to herself; 'and this is a wild duck's; and this is a pigeon's ... And here's a moor-cock's; and this – I should know it among a thousand – it's a lapwing's. Bonny bird; wheeling over our heads in the middle of the moor. It wanted to get to its nest, for the clouds touched the swells, and it felt rain coming. This feather was picked up from the heath, the bird was not shot ... I made him promise he'd never shoot a lapwing, after that, and he didn't ...' (p. 160; cf. *Hamlet*, IV.v)

Whereas Ophelia's flowers and herbs suggest her preoccupation with sexual disgrace (deflowering), Cathy's feathers point to her lost freedom, 'flying' over the moors with Heathcliff before being shot down by Linton. Now she is, in the words of the song in Angela

Carter's *Nights at the Circus*, 'only a bird in a gilded cage', the cage of adult femininity.[30]

After the onset of her illness, the doctor fears 'permanent alienation of intellect', and for two months Cathy remains in bed with 'what was denominated a brain fever', Brontë's careful choice of words foregrounding the perceived looseness of this term.[31] Although she recovers physically, she is now, in Nelly's judgement, a 'ruin of humanity'. Her symptoms are the classic symptoms of 'moral insanity', that is, melancholy and morbid thoughts. When Linton tries to cheer her, the tears 'stream down her cheeks unheeding' and she broods incessantly on her the prospect of her own death. In the last scene in which she appears, she sits as if for a portrait of the cured/ tamed madwoman, dressed in white, draped with a shawl, her hair loose but simply combed, her expression empty but appealing:

> The flash of her eyes had been succeeded by a dreamy and melancholy softness: they no longer gave the impression of looking at the objects around her ... Then, the paleness of her face – its haggard aspect having vanished as she recovered flesh – and the peculiar expression arising from her mental state, though painfully suggestive of their causes, added to the touching interest which she awakened. (p. 193)

Cathy's spirit has gone, and Linton has been left with little more than a carcass, a body that survives just long enough to give birth to a seven months' child. The 'peculiar expression' in Cathy's eyes is all that remains to signal the cost of constructing her docile pregnant body.

Cathy's illness thus passes through the two stages of insanity outlined by Thomas Graham, the first expressive of mental disturbance and disorder, the second characterised by passive melancholy. Brontë's vivid delineation of these phases suggests the strong explanatory power of the category of the 'insanity of pregnancy' in the nineteenth century. Developing out of the doctrine of maternal impressions, and constructed in response to observation (by Esquirol, Pritchard and others) of disturbed patterns of behaviour among pregnant women, the disease offered, as it were, a repertoire of symptoms for the expression of dis-ease in pregnancy. Once the disease had been named and its symptoms designated, it provided a culturally acceptable form for the expression of degrees of resistance and/or resignation to pregnancy, in a society which attempted to exert an unprecedented degree of control over women's reproductive lives.

The insanity of pregnancy is also explored in Ellen Wood's sensation novel *East Lynne* (1861). Though now, in the words of Andrew Maunder, 'one of the most famous unread works in the English language', *East Lynne* was in its day a world-wide bestseller, numbering among its fans the Prince of Wales, General Gordon, Joseph Conrad and numerous working-class men and women.[32] The insanity of pregnancy is woven into the novel's plot via the character of Lady Isobel Vane, the sensitive, high-born wife of a lawyer, Robert Carlyle. She becomes 'fanciful' and fearful during her first pregnancy, and after a difficult birth suffers from a post-partum illness in which she develops jealous obsessions about her husband. The insanity of pregnancy appears in full-blown form at the time of her 'fall', when she leaves her husband and gives birth to an illegitimate child. Before this birth, she shows symptoms of lethargy and despondency, then becomes feverish and agitated, 'panting' and threatening to lose her senses as she realises that her seducer is about to leave her. As part of her somewhat heavy-handed moral project, Wood emphasises the 'triggers' for Isobel's condition: she is (from the normative point of view, properly) stricken by remorse after her elopement and also fearful of the consequences of illegitimacy for her unborn child. However, Wood also emphasises with increasing force the hereditary component in Isobel's mental instability, the implication being that she is not fit to be a mother. Isobel's story also seems to incorporate something of Thomas Laycock's view that 'when a woman has lost her modesty, her fitness to procreate offspring of high moral excellence is probably lost too'. Her mental instability is from the first linked with a degree of moral infirmity, and it is significant that when the 'ill-starred' child of her sin is killed in a railway accident, her first feeling is 'a deep thankfulness that it had been taken so soon away from the evil to come'.[33] After her supposed death in the same accident, concerns are expressed that her only daughter may inherit her deviant tendencies. However, Isobel has returned to her marital home disguised as a governess, and it is to her, ironically, that Carlyle's second wife entrusts the moral guidance of this daughter: '"I trust you will be able to instil principles into the little girl which will keep her from a like fate"' (p. 463). The fact that the daughter suffers no ill-effects from Isobel's proximity points to the ambivalence which marks Wood's treatment of Isobel: we are meant to find her repugnant but she remains – with all her dangerous sensibility – by far the most sympathetic character in the novel.

Straightforward sympathy, rather than ambivalence, is the keynote of Elizabeth Barrett Browning's representation of the fallen woman and her pregnancy in *Aurora Leigh* (1857). In this poem, Barrett Browning solves the problem of writerly/readerly sympathy with the fallen woman by making it clear that Marian Erle has been raped while drugged and therefore cannot be held to have had any willing part in the conception of her child.[34] Barrett Browning is not quite a feminist (she thought that 'considering men and women in the mass, there *is* an *inequality* of intellect'), but she does want to speak for other women as her 'sisters'. It is thus not surprising that she depicts Marian's 'insanity of pregnancy' in vivid and affecting terms while at the same time locating her suffering firmly in a context of unjust social prejudice. Marian suffers two periods of madness, the first when, after her rape, she is left 'half-gibbering and half-raving' and is 'mad' for many weeks, wandering through the countryside with 'an awful look' on her face. There follows a calm period while she works as a servant, but then her mistress throws her out because of the pregnancy, which Marian has been too innocent to suspect. This provokes hysteria and thoughts of suicide:

> Then I rolled
> My scanty bundle up and went my way,
> Washed white with weeping, shuddering head and foot
> With blind hysteric passion, staggering forth
> Beyond those doors. 'Twas natural of course
> She should not ask me where I meant to sleep;
> I might sleep well beneath the heavy Seine,
> Like others of my sort.[35]

In Barrett Browning's reading of her situation, Marian's mental and physical sufferings are inseparable from the social structures which have produced them. It is these social structures, most notably the sexual double standard, which are the primary focus of other nineteenth-century texts dealing with illegitimate pregnancy.

'Take Your Son, Sir!'

In the late eighteenth and early nineteenth centuries, illegitimacy was discussed and represented in a range of social class contexts, involving, for example, aristocratic women becoming pregnant by their social inferiors, or middle-class women using pregnancy by a wealthier man as a lever for social advancement. In the Victorian period, however, discourses of illegitimacy tended to focus on a far more specific set of circumstances. The major focus of concern was pregnancy which resulted from the seduction of a working-class girl by a wealthy and/or aristocratic man. Such concern had a specific social context. In 1834 the New Poor Law had established sex-segregated workhouses for the indigent and had removed the right of unmarried mothers to claim financial support from the fathers of their children. Previously, such claims could have been made simply by swearing an affidavit against the man in question: he could then choose to marry the woman or give her an allowance for the support of the child. The New Poor Law met with considerable opposition, and in 1844 the so-called bastardy clauses were amended in the Little Poor Law. However, it remained far more difficult for unmarried girls and women to claim maintenance than in the past. Opposition to the bastardy clauses was based in part on their unfairness to women, in part on the widespread perception that they gave the male aristocracy a licence to rape the poor. As Barbara Taylor has suggested, such sexual rape could be seen as a metaphor for the economic rape of the poor by the rich.[36]

Such cases of illegitimacy were also commonly represented as resulting from the movement of the rural poor to manufacturing towns. In part, this reflected the reality of the large-scale migration to the towns associated with the industrial revolution. However, it also meant that in terms of representational codes, the fall of the woman could be mapped onto wider cultural polarities associated with the country and the city. Prior to her fall she could be associated with natural innocence and health, after with corruption and consequent mental and physical disease. Particular professions were also associated with the fallen woman, most notably those of the milliner and seamstress. Such professions were linked with female sexual vanity, though the vanity they served was not that of the workers but of their wealthy female clients: it was claimed in some Victorian treatises that 'love of finery' was a major cause of prostitution.

Elizabeth Gaskell's novel *Ruth* (1853) was an extremely influential representation of illegitimate motherhood. The story was loosely based on a girl Gaskell encountered in her charitable work, who was neglected by her mother, placed in an orphanage and then became a dressmaker's apprentice. Through an almost incredible series of misfortunes, she was seduced by her doctor, who turned up again after she was imprisoned, as the prison doctor.[37] Like the girl Gaskell worked with, Ruth comes from a respectable home and like her she 'falls' as a result of a series of unfortunate coincidences. The main difficulty in the novel is the question of Ruth's guilt, on which Gaskell insists despite the fact that she also represents Ruth as unfailingly gentle and virtuous. From the warm reviews the book received it would seem that the Victorian public might have been prepared to countenance the argument, implicit in the novel, that in cases such as this the young girl who has been seduced might be almost entirely blameless. However, either Gaskell was convinced that Ruth's lapse represented an absolute sin, or she was too fearful of the reviewers and public to make that case. As a result, the construction of the character of Ruth remains contradictory. As W.R. Greg put it in an article in *The National Review*, Gaskell has described a lapse from chastity 'as faultless as such a fault can be; and then, with damaging and unfaithful inconsistency, has given in to the world's estimate in such matters'.[38]

Gaskell follows contemporary representations of the fallen woman in giving Ruth a country childhood which figures prelapsarian innocence and ignorance.[39] She has grown up in a farmhouse which Gaskell presents in terms of an ideal, organic domesticity: the house gives 'a full and complete idea of a "Home." All its gables and nooks were blended and held together by the tender green of the climbing roses and young creepers.'[40] However, Ruth's parents' deaths and the carelessness of a guardian conspire to bring her to work as a seamstress in the local town, where she suffers from poverty, cold and hunger. Here Gaskell's account dovetails with contemporary representations of the seamstress, who was commonly depicted as pale and overworked, the harsh conditions of her existence often leading to illness and premature death, or alternatively to prostitution and the birth of 'unhealthy and miserable offspring'. As Deborah Cherry has shown, the image of the seamstress took hold in the popular imagination as *the* representative of the working woman, provoking ambivalent responses.[41] The poverty and overwork associated with such women inspired pity, but there was anxiety too about the possibility that such 'unnatural' work (often taking place during night hours, in a reversal of the natural order), could create 'disordered' female bodies.

Gaskell thus locates Ruth in what had become a familiar context, but from the first stresses her exceptionality. Ruth is sensitive, discriminating and beautiful; she is also extremely 'innocent' – in other words, she knows nothing of conventional sexual morality or of the workings of her own body. She is unaware that she has become pregnant until after her seducer has abandoned her, when her distress leads to a fever and a medical examination. Her reaction to the news ties in with the ideological burden of the novel: she thanks God as though for a blessing and vows to be 'so good'. *Ruth* endorses and re-presents much of the contemporary ideology of maternity which was expressed in such works as Sarah Lewis's *Woman's Mission* (1839) and Sarah Stickney Ellis's *The Mothers of England: Their Influence and Responsibility* (1843). In a representative passage, Lewis argued that 'the most powerful of all moral influences is the maternal. On the maternal character depends the mind, the prejudices, the virtues of nations; in other words the regeneration of mankind.'[42] Gaskell, accordingly, constructs Ruth as a sinner who is given not only the means of her own redemption through repentance, but also the opportunity to bring another 'soul' to goodness through virtuous maternal influence. Ruth dedicates herself to this double project, which begins even before her child's birth, and is represented metaphorically by her adoption of 'the coarsest linen, the homeliest dark blue print' for her own clothes, while she converts the fine linen given to her by her lover into 'small garments, most daintily stitched and made ready for the little creature, for whom in its white purity of soul nothing could be too precious' (pp. 158–9). This is an image which encodes a number of transformations. The fine cloth which has been the wages of sin is converted a signifier of purity and (re)birth. Ruth also turns the trade which was the means of her fall into a means of redemption, sewing for her child and later for her living. Her actions in reserving the coarse cloth for herself and stitching fine linen for her child also figure the maternal sacrifices she makes. These sacrifices are material and emotional, and perhaps even, in pregnancy, physiological. Gaskell seems to hint here at the 'parasitical' model of pregnancy whereby the mother was thought to sacrifice her own health and devote all her physical resources to the development of the 'little creature'.

While Gaskell's novel reflects and endorses many aspects of contemporary ideology, particularly in relation to maternity, it also takes issue with some widely held beliefs. Gaskell challenges the idea of women's 'natural' purity, for example, showing that innocence and purity are not enough to protect women. It is Ruth's ignorance which leads to her fall, and she certainly possesses no feminine 'second nature' which will rescue her from danger. Belonging as she did to middle-class reforming circles, Gaskell is also extremely critical of contemporary attitudes to 'fallen women' which would exclude them from virtuous society for fear of moral contagion. The vocabulary of physical disease transmission was frequently mobilised in such contexts and in Gaskell's novel the bigoted and tyrannical businessman Bradshaw expresses the hope that his children have not been 'contaminated' by their association with Ruth (p. 340). Gaskell undercuts such ideas, for it turns out to have been rather the reverse: Ruth's pure affection has been an influence for good in Bradshaw's household, while his narrow utilitarianism has led his son into financial misconduct. Gaskell's main target, however, is the sexual double standard, which she highlights in a plot twist which brings Ruth's seducer Bellingham back into her life. An interview between the two vividly dramatises the different effects of seduction on men and women, particularly if, like Ruth, the woman bears 'the badge of her shame' in the shape of a child. Bellingham has been unmarked by the affair and has continued to lead a libertine life while remaining entirely respectable – indeed, he meets Ruth again in the course of a successful campaign for election to Parliament. Ruth's life, by contrast, has been changed irreparably, and although she has (in the terms of the novel) worked through her sin to redemption, she will always bear the marks of her suffering. As she tells Bellingham:

'We are very far apart. The time that has pressed down my life like brands of hot iron, and scarred me for ever, has been nothing to you. You have talked of it with no sound of moaning in your voice – no shadow over the brightness of your face; it has left no sense of sin on your conscience, while me it haunts and haunts; and yet I might plead that I was an ignorant child – only I will not plead anything, for God knows all –' (pp. 302–3)

Yet though Gaskell is strongly critical of the double standard, the novel retains its contradictions. For example, there is a sub-textual sense of sexual shame which seems to drive the novel's conclusion, in which Ruth dies of fever after nursing Bellingham. Such a purgatorial ending was queried even by such a (relatively) conservative commentator as Charlotte Brontë, who demanded of Gaskell, 'Why should she die? Why are we to shut up the book weeping?'

There is a marked contrast between *Ruth* and *Adam Bede* (1859), the other major novel of this period to tackle the question of illegitimate pregnancy. From the first, Ruth welcomes 'the strange, new, delicious prospect of becoming a mother' (p. 26) and, as we have seen, Gaskell's novel is strongly focused on the redemptive power of maternal love. George Eliot's novel was conceived as a riposte to and a rewriting of *Ruth*, and offers a very different take on the question of maternal feeling. For Gaskell, maternal love was natural, even though she recognised that it might wither or be corrupted in difficult circumstances. The majority of contemporary commentators concurred, with even radical campaigners such as Josephine Butler arguing that 'the maternal character' was 'deeply rooted' in almost all women: 'It will always be in her nature to foster, to cherish, to take the part of the weak.'[43] The project of *Adam Bede*, however, is to demonstrate that maternal feeling is a social construction and to show too that a failure to recognise this is damaging to women and men alike. Eliot breaks the links between biological femininity and the construction of mother-love through her treatment of Hetty Sorrel, who is, importantly, presented as a physiologically perfect specimen of young womanhood, a 'springtide beauty'. Yet despite her marked biological femininity, Hetty has no maternal instinct. She dislikes looking after her aunt's children, thinking of them as 'buzzing insects' sent to plague her, and 'would have been glad to hear that she should never see a child again; they were worse than the nasty little lambs that the shepherd was always bringing in'.[44] A good deal of textual effort is expended on considering the causes of this 'unnatural' quality, which Eliot places in the context of a profoundly cultural understanding of the formation of identity. Hetty is not maternal because she has not developed a sense of the existence of others. The suggestion is that she has been unable to reach such an understanding because her uncle and aunt have never penetrated to her inner life. Mrs Poyser has taught Hetty 'everything as belongs to a house' and has 'told her her duty often enough', but has not cared to investigate Hetty's feelings or hopes (p. 153). Hetty's childlike appearance has also encouraged others to treat her as not quite an adult, not quite real. In effect, she has been infantilised and treated as a pretty surface: no wonder that she is childlike and shallow.

Hetty's lack of maternal instinct is (paradoxically, in view of its tragic effects) linked with the higher stage of development reached by human beings in comparison with other animals. 1859 was the year in which Darwin's *Origin of Species* was published, and Eliot pursues the evolutionary question in *Adam Bede* through the recurrent motif of Bartle Massey's dog.[45] As village schoolmaster Bartle is the representative of culture and his dog Vixen is the representative of female nature. Bartle always refers to Vixen as a woman, and projects his curmudgeonly view of women onto her. Thus when he feeds her he comments, '"She'll do nothing with it but nourish those unnecessary babbies. That's the way with these women – they've got no head pieces to nourish, and so their food all runs either to fat or to brats."' This, of course, does no more than reflect the views of contemporaries like Herbert Spencer (with whom Eliot had had a romance), who argued that women were formed primarily for reproduction. Yet in a significant additional comment, Bartle asks in relation to Vixen,

'"Where's the use of talking to a woman with babbies? ... she's got no conscience – no conscience – it's all run to milk!"' (p. 243). Although Bartle here confounds women and animals, the text does not. Hetty does not merely follow blind instinct: she is driven by culturally constructed feelings of ambition, guilt and shame to abandon her child. She is thus suspended uneasily between mere animal life and the more sophisticated forms of consciousness exhibited in the novel, most notably by her cousin Dinah, the Methodist preacher.

Eliot's treatment of Hetty's experience of pregnancy is both searching and broadly sympathetic.[46] Hetty's immediate response is like that of the girls described in William Hunter's treatise on infanticide, which Eliot may have known: it is one of confusion and denial. When she first realises that she may be pregnant, she waits 'in the blind vague hope that something would happen to set her free from her terror' and thinks that 'something *must* happen' to set her free from dread (p. 366). All her efforts then become concentrated on disguise. Her successful concealment from her family of a five or six months' pregnancy is explained by the narrator in terms of the 'familiar unsuspecting eye' leaving unnoticed what 'the stranger's eye detects' (p. 378). However, as Leigh Summers has pointed out, in the nineteenth century corsetry offered 'an almost undetectable method of disguising pregnancy', especially if the foetus was small.[47] Certainly, the narrator's repeated comments on Hetty's dressing to conceal her condition hint, however covertly, at the use of corsetry. It is impossible to determine how far Eliot was thinking in terms of historical accuracy here (*Adam Bede* was set back at a distance of sixty years), but some form of home-made corset would have been worn by a woman of Hetty's class at the turn of the century, as well as in the mid-Victorian period. The use of corsets during pregnancy was routinely condemned in advice books for women. In his hugely popular *Advice to a Wife on the Management of her Own Health and on the Treatment of Some of the Complaints Incidental to Pregnancy, Labour, and Suckling* Henry Chavasse claimed (probably correctly) that the use of corsets encouraged uterine prolapse.[48] He, like others, also emphasised the dangers posed to the foetus by corsetry, which included prematurity: Eliot may have had this in mind as one cause of the premature birth of Hetty's child.

Once concealment of her pregnancy is no longer possible, Hetty sets out in search of her seducer, the young squire Arthur Donnithorne. She knows that he will not marry her, but she clings to the idea of his 'receiving her tenderly'. She has reached the stage described by Hunter: 'In proportion as she loses the hope either of having been mistaken with regard to pregnancy, of being relieved from her terrors by a fortunate miscarriage, she every day sees her danger nearer and nearer, and her mind more overwhelmed by terror and despair.'[49] Hetty's journey through pregnancy becomes a kind of reverse pilgrimage, in which she loses 'all love and belief in love' and becomes prey to suicidal thoughts. We are invited to pity her condition, but the narrator underlines the fact that her suffering is the greater because of her moral failings. In marked contrast to Ruth, the pregnant Hetty has no thought of her unborn child, nor of her responsibility for it: 'Poor wandering Hetty, with the rounded childish face, and the hard unloving despairing soul looking out of it – with the narrow heart and narrow thoughts, no room in them for any sorrows but her own, and tasting that sorrow with the more intense bitterness!' (p. 391). The birth of her child does nothing to change this, as we learn from her confession to her cousin Dinah. What the birth means to Hetty is the possibility of freedom, as she conceives the idea of abandoning the child and returning to her home: 'I thought I should get rid of all my misery, and go back home, and never let 'em know why I ran away' (p. 457). This regressive fantasy is entirely in line with what we know of Hetty's character. However, Eliot softens the representation of infanticide by attributing some minimal maternal feelings to Hetty. She is haunted by her child's cries after she has buried it in grass and woodchips, and her mental confusion and physical exhaustion are also emphasised. As an intervention in contemporary debates about infanticide, *Adam Bede* is clearly on the side of compassion for abandoned mothers who faced social opprobrium and the loss of life-opportunities.[50]

None the less, and in marked contrast to *Ruth*, the novel makes no explicit comment on the sexual double standard. In part, this can be ascribed to the fact that Eliot's realist aesthetic was founded on the patient teasing out of particular relationships and sets of circumstances: she was averse to generalisations about social issues. As the novel has a male narrator, the elision of the issue is also consistent with the novel's narrative perspective. None the less, it is striking that there is no comment on the obvious disproportion between the suffering and punishment of Hetty and Arthur. If anything, Eliot seems to wish to refer their respective fates to differences in their character. Arthur is a social being with a 'loving nature': his kindnesses are pithily described as 'the common issue of his weaknesses and good qualities, of his egoism and his sympathy' (p. 313). Sympathy throughout Eliot's work is *the* redeeming virtue, and it is the one quality Hetty absolutely lacks. Yet the differences between Arthur's and Hetty's fates are clearly the result of wider social forces, regardless of character. It is these pressures which drive Hetty to infanticide, followed by her public trial and transportation, topped off by her death when she is finally returning home to England. Arthur lives, though somewhat impaired in health, to be welcomed back into his community and his role as squire.

Eliot's reticence on this issue can be attributed above all to her reluctance to have her worked judged with reference to her gender. Hence her use of a male pseudonym and, in this first novel, of a male narrator. She shies away from any special pleading on behalf of women, to the point of positioning infanticide as a crime which could be associated with men as much as women. In the extraordinary passage in which Hetty is first introduced to the reader, Eliot smoothly incorporates into the narrative voice male sadistic fantasies directed towards women *and* babies:

> there is one order of beauty which seems made to turn the heads not only of men, but of all intelligent mammals, even of women. It is a beauty like that of kittens, or very small downy ducks making gentle rippling noises with their soft bills, or babies just beginning to toddle and to engage in conscious mischief – a beauty with which you can never be angry, but that you feel ready to crush for inability to comprehend the state of mind into which it throws you. (p. 81)

Eliot's acknowledgement of the fact that a man might feel compelled to 'crush' a baby because of the uncontrollable emotions it inspired in him not only foretells Hetty's crime, but simultaneously places it in a context wider than that of infanticide by women. Eliot thus deflects attention way from infanticide as a gender issue. Although *Adam Bede* interrogates the ideology of maternal love, it stops short of a critique of the social codes and structures which endorse and exacerbate the sexes' asymmetrical relationship to reproduction.

Although Victorian painters, and in particular the Pre-Raphaelites, were also interested in the 'fallen woman', visual representations of pregnancy are rare in this period. An exception is Ford Madox Brown's painting 'Take Your Son, Sir!', which can be read alongside Gaskell's *Ruth* as a polemic engaging with the double standard. The models for the painting were Brown's second wife, Emma, and their three-month-old son. The painting was begun in 1851 and went through several stages, before being left unfinished around 1856–7. The title points to Brown's intention that it should be read in terms of the seduction of a servant by the portly master reflected in the mirror behind her. The pose of the woman, her eyes raised to engage with the spectator, implies supplication, but the rendering of the child, emerging as though being pulled out of the womb, has a very different effect. Brown makes direct reference here to the visual conventions of the obstetrical textbook and medical text. The folds of the mother's dress in the painting mirror the representation of the placenta and lining of the womb in Rymsdyk's engravings for Hunter and Smellie, and the dangling folds of the drapery on the lower left and right mimic the representation of the fallopian tubes and uterine vessels. Further, the mother's finger, grasping the child's leg and resting on the navel, suggests the umbilical cord, which reappears in the small snake of drapery by the child's left hand. In merging a clothed and respectable female figure with an image drawn from the obstetrical atlas, Brown emphasises the contrast between surface decorum and the painful realities of seduction, birth and death, and thus issues a challenge to the duplicity of Victorian society. The obstetric image has a powerful charge, for it suggests the potential pathologies of pregnancy and childbirth, and also carries overtones of mortality from its association with morbid anatomy.

The lack of visual images of pregnancy in this period must be due, in large part, to the extraordinarily powerful taboo surrounding the subject in middle-class circles. It has been argued by Judith Lewis that throughout the nineteenth century, aristocratic women continued to live an active social life during their pregnancies.[51] The letters of Queen Victoria seem to bear this out. In March 1870, for example, she wrote:

> And now one of the new fashions of our very elegant society is to go in perfectly light-coloured dresses – quite tight – without a particle of shawl or scarf ... and to dance within a fortnight of their confinement and even valse at seven months!!! Where is delicacy of feeling going to?[52]

In middle-class circles, by contrast, pregnancy was too delicate a subject to be discussed in mixed company. Pregnant women concealed their increasing size with voluminous clothes, with draperies such as the shawl and scarf recommended by Queen Victoria, and, of course, with corsetry. Their social life was also restricted in late pregnancy, ostensibly on the grounds of health but more probably because of the greater visibility of their condition. The sources of this taboo/shame are complex and its strength in this period surprising, given that there was on the

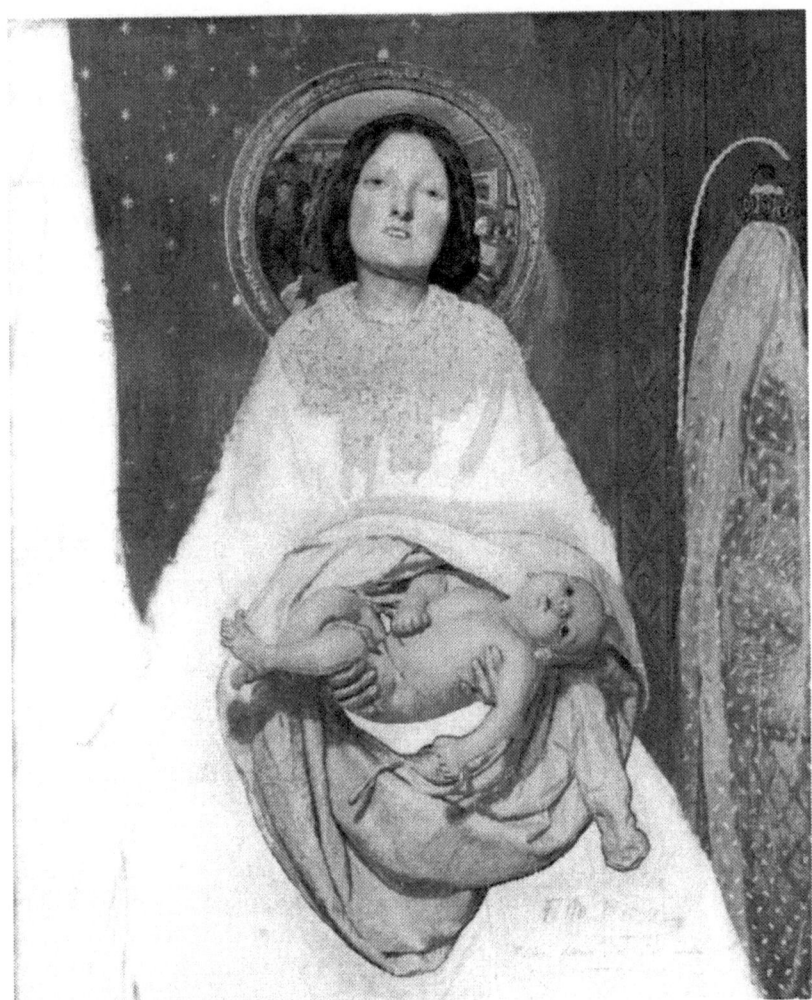

Figure 4   Ford Madox Brown 'Take Your Son, Sir!', c.1857 (detail). Courtesy of Tate London.

throne a woman who herself bore nine children between 1839 and 1857. However, this fact may itself have been one of the major contributing factors. Historians have often noted Queen Victoria's strong identification with middle-class values, and in relation to pregnancy her attitudes both reflected and, more importantly, influenced those of her middle-class subjects. Her letters to her daughter reveal her sense of pregnancy as both a physical imposition and a psychological constraint. In one letter she writes:

> to reply to your observation that you find a married woman has much more liberty than an unmarried one; in one sense of the word she has, – but what I meant was – in a physical point of view – and if you have hereafter (as I had constantly for the first 2 years of my marriage) – aches – and sufferings and miseries and plagues – which you must struggle against – and enjoyments etc. to give up – constant precautions to take, you will feel the yoke of a married woman! ... I had 9 times for 8 months to bear with those above-named enemies and real misery (beside many duties) and I own it tried me sorely; one feels so pinned down – one's wings clipped.[53]

The metaphor of the clipped wings and caged bird echoes the metaphors used in relation to Catherine Linton in *Wuthering Heights*: Victoria, like Catherine, experienced not just physical discomfort but depression ('miseries ... real misery') and a sense of entrapment. More significantly, she experienced shame and embarrassment in relation to her pregnancies, and felt keenly the contrast between her subjection to 'animal' process and the freedom of her husband and prime ministers (who were theoretically subordinate to her). Writing to her daughter she commented, 'What you say of the pride of giving life to an immortal soul is very fine, dear, but I own I cannot enter into that; I think much more of our being like a cow or a dog at such moments; when our poor nature becomes so very animal and unecstatic.' In the same letter, she stressed the importance of 'delicacy' and went on to describe her own embarrassment and dislike of being looked at when she first became pregnant: 'Think of me who at that first time, very unreasonable, and perfectly furious as I was to be caught, having to have drawing rooms and levees and made to sit down – and be stared at and take every sort of precaution.'[54] In another letter she comments: 'I positively think those ladies who are always enceinte quite disgusting; it is more like a rabbit or guinea pig than anything else and really it is not very nice.'[55]

Victoria's comments both reflect and endorse a cultural framing of the female pregnant body as animalistic, even grotesque. Mary Russo has described the grotesque body as 'open, protruding, irregular, secreting, multiple, and changing' and as connected with social transformation.[56] In screening the pregnant body, middle-class Victorian society sought to disavow, perhaps, not only female sexuality, but also the possibilities of social transformation which might be connected with it.

3
Mothering the Race

Degeneration and eugenic feminism

In the last two decades of the nineteenth century, reproduction became a highly political issue as it became closely entwined with concerns about the Empire. For the first time in centuries the birth rate was falling: from 153.5 births per 1,000 women aged 15–44 in 1876–80 to 105.3 in 1906–10. At the same time, infant mortality remained relatively high and, if anything, was increasing. Average mortality for the decade 1890–1900 was 154 per 1,000 live births; it had been 142 per 1,000 live births in the 1880s.[1] Commentators at the time agreed that 'population was power' in the context of a nation-state struggling with other nations for imperial control, and there was real concern that the Empire could not be maintained without 'the power of a white population, proportionate in numbers, vigour and cohesion to the vast territories which the British democracies in the Mother Country and the Colonies control'.[2] Not only was the nation not maintaining its stock, but it was feared that the quality of that stock was declining. The Boer War (1899–1902) brought this second issue into sharp focus. In 1899, a third of the recruits who offered themselves for military service were rejected as unfit. After the war, an influential article by General John Frederick Maurice, entitled 'Where to Get Men', described the parlous state of health of the nation's young men and stimulated the setting up of an Interdepartmental Committee to look into the question of 'the Physical Deterioration of the Population'.[3] In its Report (1904), the inquiry refuted many of Maurice's claims, arguing that his statistics were untrustworthy, but it did make recommendations for the improvement of the nation's health. These included the compilation of more reliable statistics in relation to health in pregnancy and childbirth.

The preoccupation with the quality and quantity of the nation's stock was linked not only with concerns about maintaining the Empire, but also with the complex racial anxieties associated with the imperial project. The precise meaning in this period of the term 'race' (or, as it often appeared, 'Race') is difficult to pin down. Sometimes its use is almost interchangeable with the nation, sometimes it refers to wider groupings, as in the 'Anglo-Saxon race'.[4] Implicit in contemporary discussions is the assumption, underpinned by eugenic thought, that white Europeans were the most highly developed of all races.

Eugenics had its origins in the work of Francis Galton, who developed his ideas about the inheritance of superior mental qualities after reading his cousin Charles Darwin's *Origin of Species*. Galton took the view that the quality of a race could be judged by the frequency with which it produced men of 'high natural ability': according to him, white Europeans scored highly in this respect and were thus destined to sweep away less gifted races. However, this natural process could be deliberately accelerated, and, as part of the imperial project, Galton recommended a process of controlled selection whereby the breeding of the superior race would be encouraged and that of inferior races gradually discouraged. He describes his 'merciful' approach to racial eugenics in these terms:

> Whenever a low race is preserved under conditions of life that exact a high level of efficiency, it must be subjected to rigorous selection. The few best specimens of that race can alone be allowed to become parents, and not many of their descendants can be allowed to live. On the other hand, if a higher race be substituted for the low one, all this terrible misery disappears. The most merciful form of what I ventured to call 'eugenics' would consist in watching for the indications of superior strains or races, and in so favouring them that their progeny shall outnumber and gradually replace that of the old one.[5]

While Galton was optimistic about the eventual dominance of the European race, many were fearful of what became known as 'race deterioration'. Max Nordau's influential *Degeneration* (1895) fuelled such fears by introducing the concept of 'noxious influences' which would create a degenerate 'sub-species'. Such a sub-species would possess 'the capacity of transmitting to its offspring, in a continuously increasing degree, its peculiarities, these being morbid deviations from the normal form – gaps in development, malformations and infirmities'. The causes of degeneracy, according to Nordau, were addiction to narcotics and stimulants, the ingestion of tainted foods and the prevalence of 'organic poisons' such as syphilis and tuberculosis. Although Nordau argued that degenerates would ultimately breed themselves out of existence, his book provoked anxiety and stimulated a public debate because the 'causes' he highlighted were so clearly visible in the modern world.[6] They can be divided into environmental factors (low-quality, industrially produced food; opiate and tobacco consumption) and hereditary ones (syphilis, tuberculosis and alcoholism were all thought to be hereditary). Of all these, syphilis caused the most concern, so that even a moderate commentator like J.W. Ballantyne was spurred into rhetorical mode when he came to consider the effects of syphilis on the unborn child. In his book *Expectant Motherhood* (1914), he wrote that syphilis brings long-continued disease to the mother and is a 'death warrant' for the unborn child: 'even if the syphilitic child in the womb comes into the world alive, it is already tainted, and lives its whole life, short or long, under the black shadow of a malady which may attack every tissue in the body and weaken every function both of body and mind.'[7]

The influence of eugenics extended not only to issues of race but also to those of class. The emphasis on class was distinctively British and derived from Galton's view that pauperism was genetic, caused by inherited defect rather than by social and environmental conditions. In an 1891 paper he argued that 'the race' could be improved by differential breeding, an argument which was enthusiastically taken up by the Eugenics Education Society, founded in 1907. The Society funded so-called 'pauper pedigree studies' which were designed to document the transmission of undesirable characteristics. Two such studies formed part of the Society's submission to the Committee on Poor Law Reform in 1910. They were accompanied by a commentary listing the 'inherent defects' to be found among pauper families:

> The Committee is quite clear that the paupers whom they have seen and examined individually are characterised by some obvious vice or defect such as drunkenness, theft, persistent laziness, a tubercular diathesis, mental deficiency, deliberate moral obliquity or general weakness of character, manifested by want of initiative or energy or stamina.[8]

The fact that this list of 'defects' overlapped so closely with Nordau's signs of 'degeneration' indicates the strength of the belief that the poorer classes constituted a threat to and a drag on the whole of society.

This emphasis on differential breeding formed a context too for 'eugenic feminism'. The relationship between feminism and eugenics was complicated by the conflict which arose in the later nineteenth century between women's demand for increased access to education and the view, put forward by earlier writers such as Herbert Spencer and advanced with increasing frequency by medical commentators, that such education was incompatible with healthy reproduction. Henry Maudsley, for example, had put the case against women's education in 1874 in an article in the *Fortnightly Review* in which he argued: 'It will have to be considered whether women can scorn delights, and live laborious days of intellectual exercise and production, without injury to their functions as the conceivers, mothers, and nurses of children.'[9] Elizabeth Garrett Anderson's tart response, in an article which appeared the following month, was that 'when we are told that in the labour of life women cannot disregard their special physiological functions without danger to health, it is difficult to understand what is meant, considering that in adult life healthy women do as rule disregard them almost completely'.[10]

The view that intellectual work compromised women's reproductive health held most sway in America, where it was promoted by S. Weir Mitchell, the influential physician who treated the novelist Charlotte Perkins Gilman for postnatal depression. Mitchell argued that too much study during puberty endangered 'future womanly usefulness', and that in adult life 'the matured man certainly surpasses the woman in persistent energy and capacity for unbroken brain-work. If then she matches herself against him, it will be, with some exceptions, at bitter cost'.[11]

The position of the eugenicists was that women should not be encouraged to develop qualities, such as intellectual power and great athletic strength, which were incompatible with motherhood. They should also prioritise the choosing of a mate over the desire for a role in social or public life. While we might expect that feminists would be hostile to such ideas, in practice there were many ways in which eugenic thought could be used to support, or at least complement, feminist demands. Issues of maternal and child welfare were central for many feminists in this period, and in this area feminists and eugenicists might have common goals, even if they came to them from very different perspectives. Moreover, eugenicists like Caleb Williams Saleeby attempted to mediate between feminism and eugenics by making a flattering appeal to 'the best women' to reproduce for the benefit of the race. In his *Woman and Womanhood: A Search for Principles* (1912), he coined the term 'eugenic feminism' in connection with his ardent belief that *'the best women must be the mothers of the future'* (original emphasis). He went on to suggest:

> To-day, the natural differences between individuals of both sexes, and the importance of their right selection for the transmission of their characters to the future, are clearly before the minds of those who think at all on these subjects. On various occasions I have raised this issue between Feminism and Eugenics, suggesting that there are varieties of feminism, making various demands for women which are utterly to be condemned because they not merely ignore eugenics, but are opposed to it, and would, if successful, be therefore ruinous to the race.[12]

Such arguments were accepted by many feminists, including Marie Stopes, best remembered for establishing the first birth control clinic in 1921. Stopes was connected with the Eugenics Education Society, and in the two books she published in 1918, *Married Love* and *Wise Parenthood*, she argued, in line with Saleeby's position, that the healthy and gifted had a duty to rear children for the good of the race:

> Whatever theory of the transmission of characteristics scientists may ultimately adopt, there can be little doubt in the minds of rational people that heredity *does* tell, and that children who descend from a double line of healthy and intelligent parents are better equipped to face whatever difficulties in their environment may later arise than are children from unsound stock. As Sir James Barr said in the *British Medical Journal*, 1918: 'There is no equality in nature among children nor among adults, and if there is to be a much-needed improvement in the race, we must breed from the physically, morally and intellectually fit.'[13]

None the less, like many feminists, Stopes distanced herself from some aspects of eugenic thought. In her view no woman, however healthy and gifted, should be required to spend years of her life breeding. In *Radiant Motherhood* she argued that the best woman was the one who, 'out of a long, healthy and vitally active life, is called upon to spend but a comparatively small proportion of her years in an *exclusive* sub-servience to motherhood'. If women devoted themselves entirely to reproduction, this would merely create 'an endless chain of fruitless lives all looking ever to some supreme future consummation which never materializes'.[14]

An early 'New Woman' novel which reflects anxieties about degeneration and simultaneously promotes a eugenic agenda is Sarah Grand's *The Heavenly Twins* (1893).[15] The novel's concern with these issues is signalled by epigraphs taken from Charles Darwin: in one Darwin expresses his agreement with Galton that 'most of our qualities are innate', and in another notes that 'the struggle between the races of man' depends 'entirely on intellectual and *moral* qualities'. Grand pursues the issue of syphilis and degeneration through the figure of Sir Mosley Mentieth, one of a group of dissolute young officers. When he first appears in the novel the narrator compares him to an ape, thus calling up the shadow of degeneration, or evolution running backwards. He is also described as one of the representatives of 'old English houses that once brought men of notable size and virile [*sic*] into the world, but are now only equal to the production of curious survivals, tending surely to extinction like the elephant, and by an analogous process'.[16] However, Mentieth's syphilitic 'tendency to extinction' naturally involves others. He marries an innocent young girl who contracts the disease from him and communicates it to their child, born within a year of their marriage. The narrator links the disease with exhaustion and extinction in a description of Edith's relation to her child:

> She had no smile for him, and uttered no baby words to him – nor had he a smile for her. He was old, old already, and exhausted with suffering, and as his gaze wandered from one to the other it was easy to believe that he was asking each dumbly why had he ever been born? (p. 289)

The Heavenly Twins engages not just with syphilitic degeneration, but also with the sexual double standard in relation to the disease. The novel was published seven years after the repeal of the Contagious Diseases Acts, which constituted an attempt to control the spread of venereal diseases by making it possible for women suspected of being prostitutes to be detained and medically examined for symptoms of disease. Men were excluded from the Act, a reflection of the widespread belief that gonorrhoea and syphilis could be passed only from women to men. In making it clear that Edith has contracted syphilis from Mentieth, the novel challenges gendered myths about the transmission of venereal disease, as well dispelling female ignorance about this and other sexual matters.

The novel's eugenic feminist message is expressed in a passage in which it is argued that 'all this unrest and rebellion against the old established abuses amongst women is simply an effort of nature to improve the race. The men of the present day will have a bad time if they resist the onward impulse; but, in any case, the men of the future will have good reason to arise and call their mothers blessed' (p. 219). In other words, independent, educated women, who are given the same opportunities for personal development as men, will make the best 'mothers of the race' and will make wise reproductive choices. One woman with such potential is Evadne Frayling, a friend of Edith's and the central female character in the novel. She has a mind 'of exceptional purity as well as of exceptional strength' and has spent her adolescence reading not only a wide range of novels, but also texts in political science and in anatomy, physiology and pathology. Evadne differs from Edith in that she is not ignorant of political questions or of sexual matters. Thus, when she discovers immediately after her marriage that her husband Colquhoun has a dubious sexual history, she takes steps to protect herself, refusing to live with him as his wife. They live together as friends, but the narrator makes it clear that this is at some cost to both of them. Not only does Colquhoun desire Evadne but she desires him, feeling in moments of vulnerability a 'yearning to be held close, close; to be kissed till she could not think; to live the intoxicating life of the senses only' (p. 344). She subdues these feelings, however, and in a move that is implicitly connected with the repression of sexual appetite, also stops reading. Ideas become troublesome to her and she sinks into a state of mental torpor. As the narrator puts it, she has thus fallen into an 'unnatural state of celibacy with mental energy unapplied' (p. 350). From this point on, Evadne's story is filtered through the perspective of the alienist Dr Galbraith, whose narrative forms the concluding section of the book. In effect it forms a case history, which foregrounds many of the ambiguities of the relationship between doctors and their female patients.[17] Soon after Galbraith meets Evadne, he diagnoses her case as one of hysteria. Such a diagnosis accords with contemporary medical thinking, for Maudsley and others had linked hysteria with both sexual repression and with the restrictions on women's lives. Maudsley argued that the ill-effects of sexual repression were compounded by a lack of activity in women and young girls: 'the range of activity of women is so limited, and their available paths of work in life so few, compared with those which men have in the present social arrangements, that they have not, like men, vicarious outlets for feelings in a variety of healthy aims and pursuits.'[18] However, Grand makes a feminist point by extending Maudsley's notion of the 'range of activity' necessary for women to

include intellectual activity. Moreover, she highlights the sexual component implicit in the *treatment* of hysteria, and suggests that sexual
investment and transference could come from the doctor as well as the
patient: in the course of treating her, Galbraith falls in love with 'my
little lady'.

After the death of Evadne's husband he marries his patient,
confident that she is on the road to recovery despite the fact that an
eminent nerve specialist has warned him that 'the first call upon her
physical strength may set up a recurrence of the moral malady'. When
Evadne becomes pregnant the moral malady manifests itself in the
form of the insanity of pregnancy. This disease category continued to
feature in textbooks of obstetrics and midwifery until well into the
twentieth century. In W.F. Dakin's 1897 *Handbook of Midwifery*, for
example, it is described in the following terms:

> Child-bearing is known to have a particularly marked influence in
> causing insanity in those women who have an hereditary taint of
> madness or of other marked neurosis ... Apprehension of the
> approaching trial, or vaguely of nothing particular, becomes some-
> times, especially in women with hereditary tendencies, or who have
> been affected previously, a settled dread, and developes [sic] into
> melancholia ... She is often apathetic, caring nothing for her usual
> interests, and despairing of everything.[19]

He adds that, in rare cases, moral aberrations and a tendency to suicide
may be present. Evadne's illness follows just such a course. In her pregnancy she becomes preoccupied by fears of hereditary disease and after
reading her husband's library books on the subject she attempts
suicide, leaving a note which reads: '"I am haunted by a terrible fear ...
I have tried again and again to tell you, but I never could ... in case of
our death – nothing to save my daughter from Edith's fate – better
both die at once"' (p. 665). Galbraith finds her in time, but although
her life and that of her child are saved, in his view her mind has been
permanently damaged. He writes that 'her moral consciousness was
suspended' and describes the damage in terms of a 'cruel obliquity' of
mind.

The novel ends with his conclusion that Evadne's 'confidence in her
fellow-creatures, the source of all mental health, had been destroyed
forever, and with that confidence her sense *of the value of life and of her
own obligations* had been also injured or distorted to a degree which
could not fail to be dangerous' (p. 678; emphasis added). The 'moral

danger' lies in the fact that Evadne cannot be brought to see suicide as a sin: paradoxically, it is her abhorrence of *sexual* immorality which has brought her to this state. *The Heavenly Twins* thus ranges across the difficulties which could face would-be 'mothers of the race' as a consequence of the sexual double-standard and also explores the social aetiology of the insanity of pregnancy. The text implies that, like hysteria, this illness was a response to the cramped and constricted nature of middle-class women's lives. Evadne has suffered in her first marriage from 'galling limitations' and has had 'no purpose for which to live and make the most of her abilities'. These are Galbraith's own observations, and yet he fails to perceive that, for a woman of Evadne's potential, bearing children to a devoted second husband might not offer quite the 'purpose' she needs – rather the reverse, as it will confirm her in her confinement, in both senses of the word. Thus while Galbraith suspects an hereditary component in Evadne's illness, he simultaneously points to its circumstantial causes.

The Heavenly Twins caused a sensation when it was first published and, perhaps for this reason, was hugely successful, selling 20,000 copies immediately and being reprinted six times in the first year.

A second New Woman writer who shot to prominence in 1893 was 'George Egerton' (Mary Chavelita Dunne). Like Grand, Egerton was a feminist who was not afraid to confront scandalous subjects, and she became famous for her frank articulation of women's sexual desires. She too tackled the issue of eugenic feminism. Her best-known short story, 'A Cross Line', opens with the central character sitting on a slope reminiscent of the 'tangled bank' invoked by Darwin in *The Origin of Species* as an image of natural selection. Egerton writes:

> She is sitting on an incline in the midst of a wilderness of trees; some have blown down, some have been cut down, and the lopped branches lie about; moss and bracken and trailing bramble, fir-cones, wild rose bushes, and speckled red 'fairy hats' fight for life in wild confusion.[20]

The character 'Gypsy' muses here on questions of heredity and race, 'the why and wherefore of their distinctive natures', and gives passionate expression to the view that women are more powerful than men in their strong instincts and lack of sentimentality. She argues that men have created a sanitised version of 'woman' which obscures the truth of their strength and lawlessness: the 'elaborately reasoned codes for controlling morals or man do not weigh a jot with us against an impulse, an instinct' (p. 28). As she is speaking here to a young man who is trying to tempt her away from her marriage, the reader expects that 'an impulse' will lead Gypsy into an affair, but the choice she makes is to stay with her husband. In part, this is because she has discovered that she is pregnant. However, Egerton makes it clear that the pregnancy is merely a happy confirmation of the wise reproductive choice she has already made. As Gypsy tells her would-be lover, it is the 'primitive' element in women which explains 'why a refined, physically fragile woman will mate with a brute, a mere male animal with primitive passions – and love him– ... why strength and beauty appeal more often than the more subtly fine qualities of mind or heart' (p. 22).

Egerton here offers a version of eugenics which is distinctive in two ways. First, she stresses the primacy of women in the process of sexual selection. Darwin had argued in *The Descent of Man* that while in the earliest periods of human history women had considerable power in selecting a mate, in more organised societies, 'the strongest and most vigorous men' would always be able to select 'the more attractive women'.[21] Throughout his work he assumes that men (unlike males of other species) are the prime movers in the process of sexual selection. Egerton offers a feminist challenge to this view, and also contests Darwin's claim that where women do have free choice, 'their choice is largely influenced by the social position and wealth of the men' (p. 609). Gypsy's husband is not as wealthy as her lover or as 'subtle', but he has the 'strength and beauty' she requires. For Egerton, feminism and eugenics are entirely compatible: in driving sexual selection and reproduction, women already are the 'mothers of the race'.

Women's rights and the antenatal environment

While the eugenics movement emphasised the importance of heredity in creating 'a healthy race', a rather different, environmental approach to foetal health was also emerging. The most important figure in this respect was J.W. Ballantyne, an Edinburgh-trained doctor whose interest in antenatal health derived from his MD research on foetal malformations. Ballantyne published two studies of antenatal pathology and therapeutics in 1902 and 1904, and insisted throughout his career on the importance of research in this area, arguing that obstetricians had scant understanding of the physiology and pathology of antenatal life. However, he also wished to intervene practically in the field of antenatal care. In 1901 he published an influential article in the *British*

Medical Journal, 'A Plea for a Pro-Maternity Hospital', in which he pointed out that there was currently no provision in hospitals for the care of pregnant women before the onset of labour. He suggested that every maternity unit should have a department or annexe dedicated to the treatment of such women. These units would be for the reception of patients

> who have in past pregnancies suffered from one or other of the many complications of gestation, or in whose present condition some anomaly of the pregnant state has been diagnosed; but in time it may be taken advantage of by more or less normal ambulants, working women for example who ought to rest during the last weeks of pregnancy, but who are unable from financial reasons to do so, and by the patients who clamour for admittance to our maternities, but who are told to come back again when the 'pains have begun'.[22]

Ballantyne's position here is characteristic of his approach to antenatal care in its emphasis on the importance of clinical diagnosis *and* the social/environmental contexts of pregnancy. His argument was that pro-maternity units would allow for the study of pathological conditions such as pre-eclampsia and thus advance clinical treatment, while at the same time they would help to address environmental factors, such as overwork and poor diet, which were known to have an adverse effect on pregnancy.[23]

Three months after the publication of Ballantyne's article, the first hospital bed for the treatment of pregnant women was endowed in the Edinburgh Royal Maternity Hospital, and named the Hamilton bed after the founder of the hospital, Alexander Hamilton. Subsequently, home visits were organised for expectant mothers who were booked in for delivery at the hospital, and by 1915 outpatient antenatal consultations had been instituted there. The concept of antenatal care had been accepted, and slowly the ideas were put into practice, if not quite in the form Ballantyne had envisaged (in-patient beds specifically for pregnant women were never instituted on a large scale). Ballantyne wanted pregnant women to be given basic advice on diet and exercise and to be tested for albuminuria (the presence of albumin in the urine, which is associated with hypertension and had been linked with pre-eclampsia in the late nineteenth century). These goals began to be met initially in the context of hospital care, then through municipally funded antenatal clinics after the passing of the Maternity and Child

Welfare Act 1918. In any event, Ballantyne's importance lay not so much in the detail of his recommendations as in his drawing attention to antenatal care as the 'Cinderella' of modern medical practice. He was also a significant figure in his resistance to eugenics. In his 1914 book *Expectant Motherhood: Its Supervision and Hygiene*, written to give mothers 'a fuller knowledge of obstetrical matters' than they could find in ordinary advice books, he describes eugenics as a 'fascinating but extremely illusory science' and argues that:

> Until the full effect of surrounding the expectant mother, and through her the unborn infant, with a healthy environment has been tried; until the possible results of sending to the child's tissues through the maternal blood the right materials in their proper proportions have been thoroughly ascertained; until it is known what influence the exclusion of all toxins and toxinic agents from the life that is before birth may have...it is foolish to propose revolutionary legislation restricting marriage and encouraging the segregation of the individuals whom their contemporaries regard as unfit for procreation. (p. xii)

As this suggests, Ballantyne's interest is in the circumstantial factors which could influence the health of the unborn child. In a suggestive turn of phrase, he argues that the mother constitutes the 'environment' of the foetus: 'Although he is hidden from sight in the womb of his mother, [the unborn child] is not beyond the influences of her environment, nay, *her body is his immediate environment*, and he is profoundly affected by it for good or evil, for health or disease; so, through her, it is practicable during the nine months of pregnancy to alter for weal or for woe the child as yet unborn' (p. xiv; emphasis added).

It is his interest in the maternal environment that leads him to challenge the eugenic movement's emphasis on heredity, as he writes of 'the immediately pre-natal influences which play upon the child, possibly with even greater effect than those which are termed hereditary' (p. xv). In arguing that the maternal environment might be as or more important than hereditary factors in determining the healthy outcome of a pregnancy, Ballantyne presciently anticipates contemporary debates about the relative importance of genetic information and the intra-uterine environment in determining foetal health.[24]

Expectant Motherhood was aimed at 'the common reader' (to borrow a term from Dr Johnson and Virginia Woolf), and offers her or him a lucid and thoughtful account of the relationship between mother and child in pregnancy. Ballantyne considers two ways of reading pregnancy. On the one hand, it can be understood as a 'prejudicial parasitism, in which the mother suffers, to some extent at least, for her gestation', as the foetus takes nourishment from her and affects the chemical processes in her body. On the other, it can be understood as a 'harmonious symbiosis', in which the mother adapts to the demands of the foetus with no adverse effects on her own health (pp. 63–4). Ballantyne broadly endorses the model of harmonious symbiosis, making the point, however, that it can lay 'rather too strong an emphasis on the advantage which the mother may be expected to derive from the symbiosis between herself and her unborn infant, and scarcely enough upon the risks she runs and the price she pays in certain circumstances'. His conclusion is that 'in the vast majority of cases pregnancy is to be regarded as a condition of health and not of disease; it is physiology and not pathology. True it is health under strain ... In not a few cases pregnancy is physiology working at so high a pressure as to be perilously near pathology; in a few cases the border-line is actually overpassed' (p. 67).

The relationship between mother and child for Ballantyne is primarily a physiological one, seen in terms of exchanges between, for example, the maternal blood and the child's tissues. His presentation of such a model in a book intended for the general reader suggests the widespread acceptance in the early twentieth century of a 'scientific' model of medicine, associated with a culture of laboratory investigation into the causes of diseases such as tuberculosis. Clinical diagnosis and treatment were now understood in terms of identifying biological or physiological causes and effects. In relation to pregnancy, this created an understanding of the relationship between mother and child which differed significantly from that which informed late eighteenth- and nineteenth-century obstetrics. The relationship is no longer seen primarily in terms of affective sympathies or 'instinctive' vital systems, but in terms of physiological and pathological connections and effects. Such a shift brought concrete benefits in antenatal care, for it directed attention towards the physical conditions of pregnancy and thus to the effects of social inequality. In Ballantyne's view, pregnancy was thus a matter not only for doctors, nurses and patients, but also for social workers, legislators and political economists: too often the 'disease' which adversely affected the pregnant woman and her child was poverty. In his own medical unit, he took in women who were not 'seriously ill' but who were without adequate food and had no home comforts: their stay in the pregnancy ward improved their health and that of their child (p. 245).

Ballantyne's approach was similar in many respects to that of another influential campaigner, Dr J.W. Sykes, best known for his connection with the St Pancras School for Mothers, founded in 1907. The St Pancras School had an influence out of all proportion to its size, becoming a model institution for the emergent infant welfare movement. Its influence was due in part to the eloquence and enthusiasm of Sykes, who was Medical Officer of Health for St Pancras, and in part to the publicity generated by prominent supporters of the school such as Mrs Humphry Ward, Lady Henry Somerset and Alys Russell. Its stated aim was to combat infant mortality by educating working-class mothers in nutrition, hygiene and domestic health: the implicit assumption was that these mothers lacked knowledge rather than resources. However, when the School opened, its first practical step was to provide food for expectant and nursing mothers, and it was the nutritional help it offered which made it an immediate success. When a book detailing the philosophy and practice of the School was published in 1907, it was, accordingly, the nutritional aspect of the work that was emphasised. In his foreword, Sir Thomas Barlow argued for the need to 'bring home directly to the conscience and intelligence of the husbands and of the community that just as four-fifths of life is conduct, so the good nutrition of the mother during pregnancy counts for four-fifths of the value of the infant's start and its chance of survival'.[25] Sykes similarly wrote that, since 1904, his work in St Pancras had been based on 'the physiological law that infant life is dependent upon the mother from nine months before birth until nine months after birth, and the mother has been made the centre round which all the agencies revolve for the protection and preservation of the health of both mother and child, *for these two are one flesh more truly even than husband and wife*' (pp. 8–9; emphasis added). Sykes' concept of the mother and child as 'one flesh' echoes Ballantyne's idea of the 'symbiosis' between mother and child in pregnancy. In a subsequent chapter on 'food for mothers', it is pointed out that poorer pregnant women tend to sacrifice their own nutrition for that of their husband and existing children. The (anonymous) author asks: 'What is the reason of this extraordinary tendency of women to starve themselves? It all turns on this, that they don't think enough of themselves. They never treat themselves, either in the home or in public affairs, as of any importance' (pp. 29–30). An example of one such case is given:

Some little while ago, a woman in this state fainted away in the out-patients' department of a London hospital. Inquiry elicited that she had had no food that day, and had been on the verge of starvation for weeks. The physician sent her to the Welcome [the School was also known as the 'Babies' Welcome and School for Mothers'] and paid for her to have dinners daily until her confinement, and very gradually, day by day, she lost the look of dead hopeless despair which haunted us all at first. (p. 37)

Here, the impoverished pregnant woman is rhetorically constructed in terms of suffering, sacrificial motherhood and thus assimilated to the bourgeois ideology of maternity as selfless devotion. Such representations were undoubtedly effective in eliciting middle-class sympathy and practical support for working-class mothers.[26] Thus while, as Anna Davin has argued, there is often a tone of class-bound condescension towards the working classes in this book, and an implication that they were inherently more feckless than the middle classes, the School's reformers were also adept and successful in maintaining a focus on the environmental rather than the 'inherent' causes of ill-health.[27]

One such reformer was the poet Anna Wickham, who began to work for the School after the birth of her first son. In a memoir, she gives an account of her reasons for getting involved which offers a challenge to the very assumptions on which the School's work was based. Wickham joined not so much to educate working-class women as to be educated by them. As she notes, because she was a solicitor's wife, it was assumed that she knew how to instruct the working classes. But, remembering the skills of her working-class grandmother, she 'thought that there might well be something that I could learn from poor working-class mothers'.[28] She goes on to describe the way in which she linked up with the School's social workers, but resisted 'the contagion' of their patronising point of view. She writes: 'I did not believe that working-class mothers had less intelligence and goodwill than middle-class mothers, and since they produced a great many children with little house room and a minimum of money, I thought they must have at least as much goodwill, and more than ordinary tenacity.' Moreover, without 'looking very deeply into sociology', as she dryly puts it, Wickham realised that conditions for poorer mothers could be improved by the provision of clean saucepans and more milk. Filling a cab with these to take to the tenements to treat cases of marasmus (wasting of the body), she 'lost caste forever with the social workers' – though no doubt not with the mothers.

Wickham's proto-socialist and anti-eugenic perspective was powerfully expressed too in a lecture written for the School in 1909–10. In this she

begins by emphasising the importance of nutrition rather than education: 'However talented and however educated a mother is, she cannot
do her work well if she is denied the necessities of her work, if she has no
food to build her child before it is born or to nourish it after its birth.'[29]
She then takes on the issue of differential breeding and allegations that
the work of the School encouraged the breeding of the 'unfit'. Alluding
to information given to her by George Bernard Shaw to the effect that
marriages in the Fabian Society produced on average only 1.5 children,
she argues that while it is true that 'the comfortable classes' are not
keeping their ranks filled up, and that 'we are getting our population
from the cottage and the tenement', this is no bad thing: 'God's poor are
doing God's work.' She goes on contest the view that the children of the
poor suffer from inherent defects and argues for the importance of
nurture and the environment in rearing healthy children:

> We know that the greater number of the children are born healthy,
> that a half-starved mother, at the sacrifice of her own body, will
> produce a finer child than we have any right to expect. And we know
> the tremendous influence of environment and nurture. If the good
> children that Providence gives to us were treated well by us, we
> should not have so much to say of decadents and failures. (p. 373)

Wickham's position is close to Ballantyne's and to that of campaigners
associated with the Women's Co-operative Guild in this early twentieth-century debate over the relative influence of nature and nurture,
genes and (maternal) environment. She also addresses these issues in
her poetry, constructing the pregnant body as a nurturing environment in 'After Annunciation', for example:

> Rest, little Guest,
> Beneath my breast.
> Feed, sweet Seed,
> At your need.
> I took Love for my lord
> And this is my reward,
> My body is good earth,
> That you, dear Plant, have birth.
>   (1915)

The Women's Co-operative Guild was founded in 1883 with the
initial aim of involving the wives of co-operative members in the

movement. Under the guidance of Margaret Llewelyn Davies, who became General Secretary in 1889, it developed into a vigorous campaigning organisation, representing more than 32,000 working women. One of its main goals was to persuade the government and local authorities to improve maternal and infant care for poorer women. It was partly as a result of pressure from the Guild that Lloyd George's National Insurance Act 1911 included 30 shillings maternity benefit, which was accepted as legally the property of the mother in 1913. However, maternity benefit (which ensured the payment of medical fees for confinement) addressed only one of the immediate problems faced by poorer mothers. The underlying issues of poverty, overwork and medical neglect remained untouched. It was to draw attention to these that in 1914 Llewelyn Davies asked members of the Guild to write to her giving an account of their experiences of pregnancy. A selection of the letters was published in *Maternity: Letters from Working Women* in 1915. The book remains an invaluable resource for understanding motherhood in this period.

One of the key arguments made by the Guild was that motherhood should be supported as part of the war effort and in his Preface to *Maternity* Herbert Samuel makes the point that mothers should be protected because, without them, 'the nation is weakened. Numbers are of importance. In the competition and conflict of civilisations it is the mass of the nations that tells.'[30] He also takes a strongly anti-eugenic stand, arguing that 'the time is past when a shallow application of the doctrine of evolution led people to acquiesce in a high infant death-rate. It was thought that it meant merely the killing off of the weak, leading to the survival of the fittest ... There are few now who do not see that the high death-rate is due, in large measure, to a bad environment; and that by keeping a bad environment you produce unfitness.' Samuel went on to make the crucial point that this situation could be remedied only through government intervention: 'The infant cannot, indeed, be saved by the State. It can only be saved by the mother. But the mother can be helped and can be taught by the State.' As a result of this intervention, circulars were sent out in 1914 and 1915 instructing local authorities to instigate schemes to help mothers. Together with Lloyd George's Insurance Act, these mark the first tentative steps towards state provision for maternity.

Though the picture painted in *Maternity* is not one of unrelieved horror, it is a bleak one. A recurring theme is that of near-starvation in pregnancy. One writer had this to say of her second pregnancy:

By that time hard work and worry and insufficient food had told on my once robust constitution, with the result that I nearly lost my life through want of nourishment, and did after nine months of suffering lose my child. No one but *mothers who have gone through the ordeal of pregnancy half starved*, to finally bring a child into the world to live a living death for nine months, can understand what it means.' (pp. 23–4; emphasis added)

As many letters reveal, these women were acutely aware of the link between poor nutrition in pregnancy and the later ill-health of their children. One writes, for example: 'The past struggle left its mark on the physique of my children. One has since died of heart disease, aged ten years; another of phthisis, sixteen years; my youngest has swollen glands, and not at all robust' (pp. 37–8). Repeatedly, women comment on the ill-effects of poor nutrition in pregnancy, fully aware that, in Ballantyne's phrase, their bodies constituted their child's environment. Many had to work during their pregnancy, which, they realised, further undermined their health. One woman described a typical situation:

When the youngest was coming my husband was out of employment, so I had to go out to work myself, standing all day washing and ironing. This caused me much suffering from varicose veins, also caused the child to wedge in some way, which nearly cost both our lives. The doctor said it was the standing and the weight of the child. I have not been able to carry a child the full time since then. (pp. 22–3)

As many pointed out, the work they did in the home during pregnancy could be just as exhausting and damaging. One described a stillbirth brought on by such work: 'The child had been killed through shock, and already showed signs of mortification. I was in a poor state of health, and struggled against my strength, looking after the children's welfare and neglecting myself. In trying to lift the washing-tub it slipped, and that was the shock; and instead of resting and having advice (which I felt I could not afford), I persevered, and that was the result' (pp. 33–4). The women's testimonies in effect move the stage of class conflict into the womb: they could not be clearer about the effects on their unborn children of poor nutrition, poverty and overwork.

In her Introduction to *Maternity*, Margaret Llewelyn Davies also highlights the number of stillbirths and miscarriages suffered by these women. Among the women who wrote to her, the number of miscarriages was 218 (15.6 per 100 live births) and the number of stillbirths 83 (5.9 per 100 live births). Taken together, these show a pre-natal death rate of 21.5 per 100 live births, as against an infant death rate of 8.7. Davies is drawing attention to the fact that among these working women, the rate of *pre*-natal death was well over twice the rate of *post*-natal (infant) death. The women's letters make clear the extent of the loss of life during pregnancy, and the debilitating and depressing effect it had on them. Many women write of their nervous despair and some of near-madness. One woman described nursing a child during her fourth pregnancy in these terms:

> The strain was fearful, and one night I felt I must sleep or die – I didn't much care which; and I lay down by her side, and slept, and slept, and slept, forgetful of temperatures, nourishment or anything else ... A miscarriage followed in consequence of the strain ... The physical pain from the eczema, and working with raw and bleeding hands, threatened me with madness. (p. 45)

Another, shedding a sombre light on the 'insanity of pregnancy', comments: 'What with worry and feeling bad, I am never surprised at hearing of an expectant mother committing suicide' (p. 57).

The contributors to *Maternity* are in no doubt about what pregnant women need: food, rest and freedom from anxiety about their other children. In her Introduction, Llewelyn Davies is astute in campaigning for these things. Playing on anxieties about the strength of the nation, she emphasises the loss to the nation's stock because of pre-natal mortality, and focuses on specific and practical ways of promoting maternal health and thus preventing such deaths. Measures recommended in the appendix include the supervision of midwives, the establishment of antenatal clinics, home visiting for expectant mothers and the confinement of sick women in hospital.

The issue which, for obvious reasons, she does not tackle is birth control. Clearly, if the campaign for maternity was being fought on the grounds that the nation needed 'mass' and 'numbers', birth control could not be part of the argument. Thus, while many of the contributors write of having used abortifacients, Llewlyn Davies argues that women have recourse to these dangerous measures only because of the intolerable strain they are under.[31] If they were better off and less exhausted, she implies, there would no longer be a need for abortion or birth control. But the letters of some mothers belie this view: one writes, 'I may say that I have disgusted some of our Guild members by advocating restrictions. I think that it is better to have a small family and give them good food and everything hygienic than to let them take "pot- luck"' (p. 115). Another writes that she 'must write and explain why I advocate educating women to the idea that they should not bring children into the world without the means to provide for them', and argues that many women lead 'wasted lives', giving birth in rapid succession to children who die through ill-health.

As the women who contributed to *Maternity* were the first to point out, they were not among the worst off in pregnancy. Many poorer women suffered far more than they did: as one contributor put it, such women's lives consisted of nothing more than 'slavery and drudgery'. In her Introduction, Llewelyn Davies emphasised the fact that suffering in pregnancy was a class issue, arguing that it was necessary

> to consider the different conditions under which the middle-class and the working-class woman becomes a mother. The middle-class wife from the first moment is within reach of medical advice which can alleviate distressing illness and confinements and often prevent future ill-health or death. During the months of pregnancy she is not called upon to work; she is well fed; she is able to take the necessary rest and exercise. At the time of the birth she will have the constant attendance of doctor and nurse, and she will remain in bed until she is well enough to get up.

The working-class woman, in contrast, was 'habitually deprived' of all these things (p. 4). In response, some concessions were made in relation to the care of working-class women. The Maternity and Child Welfare Act enabled municipal authorities to give financial aid to maternity and child welfare work. The Act was, as Ann Oakley points out, 'permissive rather than mandatory' in outlining a comprehensive maternity service, but it required every local authority to set up a maternity and child welfare committee.[32] For the first time the state, in the form of the local authority, was charged with (limited) responsibility for maternal and child welfare.

Charlotte Perkins Gilman's novel *Herland*, also published in 1915, is both far removed from and sharply relevant to the world depicted in *Maternity*. Gilman is best known today as the author of *The Yellow Wallpaper* (1892), written as an attack on the rest cure treatment for 'neurasthenia' (a general fatigue or listlessness) developed by S. Weir Mitchell. However, in the early years of the twentieth century she was better known not as a fiction writer but as the author of *Women and Economics* (1898), a wide-ranging social analysis which became a world-wide best-seller. She had an international reputation as a lecturer on social and feminist issues, and was on friendly terms with George Bernard Shaw, Beatrice and Sidney Webb and other members of the Fabian Society. Although *Herland* was initially published in Gilman's periodical *The Forerunner* and would not have reached a wide audience in Britain, it is significant as one of the first science fiction fantasies about reproduction and as a probable influence on Charlotte Haldane, whose scientific romance *Man's World* is considered in chapter 4.

Herland depicts a utopian, all-female society, into which three men intrude with the aim of conquering the inhabitants. Instead, they are variously captivated, assimilated and defeated by these formidable women. In relation to maternity (and *Maternity*), the most significant point is that this is a society in which women reproduce by parthenogenesis and in which motherhood is the most sacred of callings. The (male) narrator tells us that 'Mother-love with them was not a brute passion, a mere "instinct", a wholly personal feeling; it was – a religion', and accordingly, 'before a child comes ... there is a period of utter exaltation – the whole being is uplifted and filled with a concentrated desire for that child'.[33] Such idealisation of motherhood can cut both ways, but Gilman wants pregnancy to be seen as important work, involving the mind as well as the body, and requiring economic and social support (as Llewelyn Davies also argued). The contrast between the dire conditions described in *Maternity* and the ideal conditions of *Herland* could not be greater, but Gilman does more than simply promote a vague ideal of motherhood: she offers strong arguments against those aspects of Darwinian thought which were being used in Britain and America to justify the current low level of support for maternity. According to conservative interpreters of Darwin, the 'survival of the fittest' through natural selection was an inevitable and beneficent process whereby the strongest and most competent survived, and the weak and 'unfit' were bred out of the race. According to commentators such as Lady Barrett of the Medical Women's Federation in Britain, intervention to support the weak was 'dysgenic' in that it would impede the development of the race.[34] Such a position depended, of course, on the assumption that heredity predominated over environment in the development of human characteristics. It also relied on the rejection of Jean Baptiste Lamarck's theory of the heritability of *acquired* characteristics.

In a key exchange in *Herland*, Gilman challenges such views. The population of Herland has been controlled voluntarily. Most women choose to have only one child, and if they begin to feel the desire for another, they distract themselves by throwing themselves into hard physical work (perhaps a comic allusion to Victorian 'cures' for excessive sexual desire). Given a stable population in which there is no struggle for existence, the question arises as to whether or how such a society can 'evolve'. One of the male intruders, the belligerent Terry, cannot see how the population can improve without genetic (natural) selection. One of the women, Zava, explains that they have instead 'striven for conscious improvement':

> 'But acquired traits are not transmissible,' Terry declared. 'Weissman [*sic*] has proved that.'
> They [the women] never disputed our absolute statements, only made notes of them.
> 'If that is so, then our improvement must be due either to mutation, or solely to education,' she gravely pursued. 'We certainly have improved. It may be that all these higher qualities were latent in the original mother, that careful education is bringing them out, and that our personal differences depend on slight variations in prenatal condition.' (p. 78)

Gilman here takes issue with those like Weismann who had argued against the transmission of acquired characteristics and suggests instead that desirable characteristics can be cultivated through 'careful education' and transmitted to the next generation.[35] From this point of view, the argument for the eugenicists' *laissez-faire* attitude to social inequality falls apart. For environmentalists like Gilman, desirable characteristics are developed not primarily through genetic inheritance but through cultivation. Society thus evolves not by giving free rein to nature but by attending to nurture, and education and the environment are of paramount importance. Like Ballantyne, Sykes and the mothers in *Maternity*, Gilman stresses the importance of the environment *before* birth, suggesting that variations in 'prenatal condition' might account for variations between individuals.

However, while physicians and pro- and anti-eugenicists were considering such variations in purely physical terms, pregnancy was at this time also beginning to be approached from a psychological or psychoanalytic point of view.

Analysing pregnancy

From the start, pregnancy features as a curious sub-text in the history of psychoanalysis. The first case history, on which the method of psychoanalysis was based, was that of 'Anna O' (Bertha Pappenheim), a young woman who was treated for hysteria by Joseph Breuer from 1881 to 1882. In the account of the case published in *Studies on Hysteria* (1895), Breuer explains that the cure for Anna O's wide range of hysterical symptoms, which included paralyses and hallucinations, was found almost by accident. Breuer spent many hours listening to her and recording her symptoms, but the breakthrough came when she described under hypnosis the 'psychic events' which had precipitated a particular symptom, and was immediately relieved of it. Breuer then devoted himself to the task of letting her 'talk away' her symptoms and the case apparently came to a successful conclusion in June 1882. By this time Anna O was 'free from the innumerable disturbances which she had previously exhibited'.[36]

However, this narrative of successful treatment was soon being questioned within the psychoanalytic community. In his 1916 study *The History and Practice of Psychoanalysis* Poul Bjerre noted in relation to Anna O, 'I can add that the patient was to undergo a severe crisis in addition to what was given out in the description of the case'.[37] Carl Jung mentioned in a 1925 seminar that the case of Anna O, thought of as a brilliant therapeutic success, was nothing of the kind. His remarks were based on confidential information given by Sigmund Freud, who also told Marie Bonaparte the following story about Anna O:

> Freud's memories as reported by him during these three months of analysis [Bonaparte was in analysis with Freud]
> The 16th of December [1927], in Vienna, Freud told me the Breuer story. His wife tried to kill herself towards the end of Anna = Bertha's treatment. The rest is well known: Anna's relapse, her fantasy of pregnancy, Breuer's flight.[38]

The story of Anna's phantom pregnancy seems to have been common knowledge in psychoanalytic circles, although it was not until Ernest Jones published his biography of Freud in 1956 that the 'full story' appeared in public. Freud allegedly told Jones that Breuer had developed a strong counter-transference to his 'interesting patient', which provoked jealousy and depression in his wife. Realising this, Breuer had told Anna O – whose condition had much improved – that her treatment had to end. Jones continues:

> But that evening he was fetched back, to find her in a greatly excited state, apparently as ill as ever. The patient, who according to him had appeared to be an asexual being and had never made any allusion to such *a forbidden topic* throughout the treatment, was now in the throes of a hysterical childbirth (pseudocyesis), the logical termination of a phantom pregnancy that had been invisibly developing in response to Breuer's ministrations.[39]

Horrified by having the 'sexual nature' of Anna's illness exposed in this way, Breuer hypnotised her to calm her down and fled 'in a cold sweat'. Complicating the story further, Jones claims that Breuer then left for a 'second honeymoon' with his wife, which led to an actual pregnancy. A similar account occurs in a letter from Freud to Stefan Zweig of June 1932, in which he wrote that when Breuer was summoned back to his patient at the end of her treatment he found her 'confused and writhing in abdominal cramps. Asked what was wrong with her, she replied: "Now Dr. B's child is coming!"'[40]

There have been widespread doubts about the veracity of this story. Exhaustive studies of the Anna/Bertha case and of archive material have failed to turn up any corroborative evidence for the phantom pregnancy: the only source remains Freud himself.[41] If its veracity is in doubt, must we read the narrative as a (male) fantasy of a (female) fantasy? One thing is clear: regardless of whether the pregnancy was produced by Anna or by Freud, its existence as a fiction betrays the component of erotic transference which, as Sarah Grand recognised, was liable to infiltrate the unequal relationship between male doctor and female hysteric. More significant, however, is the way in which the pregnancy circulates in Freud's accounts as a symptom.

Phantom pregnancies were frequently discussed in contemporary obstetric texts, where they were often linked with the menopause. In his *Handbook of Midwifery* W.R. Dakin noted that: 'Such a state of things is most common about the time of menopause, especially in childless women who are anxious to become mothers ... It is rather a delusion than a mistake' (p. 71). Such comments reflect the widespread and long-held view that such pregnancies were a form of wish-fulfilment: the term 'delusion' was also used by one of the doctors who attended Joanna Southcott. What is distinctive about Freud's approach is the characterisation of pregnancy (real or imagined) as a 'forbidden topic' within the protocol of Anna O's treatment. This reflects the assimilation of pregnancy to Freud's Oedipal narrative, a narrative which a Foucauldian analysis would suggest gained a productive power precisely because Freud brought it into discourse as a taboo (or 'forbidden') subject.[42]

To summarise the Oedipus complex briefly: in Freud's account of the development of sexual identity, for both male and female children the first object of proto-sexual desire is the mother. The little boy, fearing that his illicit desire for the mother will be punished by the father with castration, represses it, knowing however that one day he will stand in the place of the father with another woman/wife. The process is more complicated for the little girl. She too must repress her desire for her mother, which she does when she discovers that, like her mother, she lacks a penis. Blaming her mother for this, she turns her desire to the father, hoping to get from him a penis, or its unconscious equivalent, a baby.

The overwhelmingly patriarchal assumptions which underpin this theory scarcely need to be pointed out. It is the product of the specific context of upper-middle-class family life in late nineteenth-century Vienna, and Freud's theories reflect the centrality in that society of the father as the representative of power and authority. Hence the (otherwise extraordinary) representation of pregnancy as a secondary and derivative function, a gift from the potent father/lover to the powerless daughter/wife. Indeed, in his account of the Oedipus complex Freud comes perilously close to depicting pregnancy in parthenogenetic terms (indeed, parthenogenetic fantasies seem to be particularly prominent in this period). Pregnancy does not seem to be the result of the union of two elements, but is understood almost exclusively in terms of desire for the phallus. The fantasy Freud attributes to Anna O could thus be read as a mirror image of his own fantasy, that women desire pregnancy as means to possess the phallus. In this sense, it could be argued that it is Freud who is the hysteric, denying the double origin of pregnancy and refusing, in Juliet Mitchell's words, to 'give up the fantasy of childhood parthenogenesis'. As Mitchell argues: 'The point at which the hysteric exists is the one where the child's belief that it can have a baby from just its own body is maintained ... In regressing to this childhood, in fantasy the hysteric gives birth to himself.'[43]

Also notable is the way Freud divorces pregnancy from its historical and material contexts. While later analysts such as Helene Deutsch and Karen Horney pay close attention to the historical and social determinants of pregnancy, Freud makes no reference to such issues as differences in family structure or in economic status.[44] His men and women exist in a private 'theatre of home', engaged in a struggle for power divorced from social context. In this battle of the sexes, pregnancy figures as a threat, weapon or promise, a floating signifier rather than a material process or event. Freud simultaneously abstracts pregnancy from particular contexts, thus denuding it of certain specific meanings, and transforms it into a general symbol, thus endowing it with an enhanced metaphorical reach and power. It is this metaphorical potential which drew the attention of writers such as D.H. Lawrence and Katherine Mansfield.

Lawrence's interest in Freud's work is well known and well documented: his treatment of pregnancy in *The Rainbow* (1915) constitutes a specific intervention in the construction of pregnancy as metaphor.[45] Whereas Freud always refers pregnancy ultimately to male power, Lawrence takes the opposite path, representing pregnancy, in fantasy at least, as a form of creativity from which men are excluded. *The Rainbow* charts the experience of pregnancy across three generations, disclosing a recurrent pattern, with variations. In the first generation, Lydia Brangwen's pregnancy threatens to annihilate her husband: 'As the months of her pregnancy went on, she left him more and more alone, she was more and more unaware of him, his existence was annulled.'[46] The pregnancy is represented almost entirely from Tom's perspective (as is the birth) and the narrative tracks across his complex, flickering responses to what he perceives as Lydia's withdrawal and self-absorption. In the description of Lydia's labour, however, Lawrence borrows from the Old and New Testaments to convey Tom and Lydia's ultimate acceptance of the double origins and determinants of pregnancy: 'Their flesh was one rock from which the life gushed, out of her who was smitten and rent, from him who quivered and yielded' (p. 75). It is this acceptance of doubleness that restores the equilibrium of their relationship.

In his treatment of Lydia's daughter Anna, Lawrence explores a more strongly narcissistic approach to pregnancy. Again, the pregnancy is presented initially from the perspective of the husband, whose strongest emotion on learning of it is fear: 'And he trembled as if a wind blew on to him in strong gusts, out of the unseen. He was afraid. He was afraid to know he was alone. For she seemed fulfilled and separate and sufficient in her half of the world' (p.179). Here the biblical references suggest forms of knowledge that are immediate and prior to language, from which Will is excluded. He sees himself as an accessory, shut out from Anna's sense of completeness in pregnancy.

Her narcissistic sense of completeness/completion is figured in her dancing, undertaken at first in secret as she lifts 'her hands and her body to the Unseen, to the unseen Creator who had chosen her', then as a kind of provocation to Will:

> Because he was in the house, she had to dance before her Creator in exemption from the man. On a Saturday afternoon, when she had a fire in the bedroom, again she took off her things and danced, lifting her knees and her hands in a slow, rhythmic exulting. He was in the house, so her pride was fiercer. She would dance his nullification. (pp. 183–4)

As the narrative perspective shifts to Anna, it confirms her repudiation of Will and her fantasy of direct access to the source of life. She takes on the omnipotence of the creator, leaving Will to experience himself as a secondary being:

> For how can a man stand, unless he have something sure under his feet? Can a man tread the unstable water all his life, and call that standing? Better give in and drown at once.
> And upon what could he stand, save upon a woman? Was he then like the old man of the sea, impotent to move save upon the back of another life? Was he *impotent, or a cripple or a defective, or a fragment*? (p. 187; emphasis added)

Anna's pregnancy thus results not only in the birth of her daughter Ursula, but in Will's (re)birth as her child. The struggle between the couple teaches Will 'to be able to be alone' and gives him a self which is not just 'a relative self'. However, in the words of the narrator, 'it was a very dumb, weak, helpless self, a crawling nursling. He went about very quiet, and in a way, submissive' (p. 190). The structure of Will and Anna's marriage is determined by this first preg- nancy, and could thus be read as a reversal of the Freudian paradigm, both partners ascribing phallic power to Anna. None the less, the narrator underlines the fact that Anna's repeated pregnancies also function as a kind of displacement activity which leads her to 'relin- quish the adventure' of her life. She becomes a liminal figure as she awaits the birth of each new child: 'She was a door and a threshold, she herself. Through her another soul was coming, to stand upon her as upon the threshold, looking out, shading its eyes for the direction to take' (p. 196).

Following the pattern of repetition with variation, Ursula struggles to establish a sense of self and resist such an absorption into maternity. She is threatened by it when she becomes pregnant with her lover's child and thinks of bringing up the child herself, but she suffers a miscarriage and is alone at the close of the novel. There is a suggestion that the failure of the pregnancy is inevitable, for it is the result of a sexual encounter which is couched in terms of a deadly struggle and ordeal: 'The fight, the struggle for consummation was terrible. It lasted till it was agony to his soul, till he succumbed, till he gave way as if dead' (p. 480). Thus Ursula's 'soul is sick' when she realises she is pregnant: 'It seemed, this child, like the seal set on her own nullity' (p. 484). At this point, there is a sense that Lawrence is overloading the dice: Ursula's pregnancy is freighted with a significance that belongs to a different, wider argument.

This is a point made by Anna Wickham in 'The Spirit of the Lawrence Women'.[47] Wickham had been friendly with Lawrence in 1914–15, but had noted at the time his 'very curious attitude to the whole subject of reproduction'. Her article seems to have been prompted by the publication of Catherine Carswell's 1932 book about Lawrence, *The Savage Pilgrimage*, for she took particular exception to a letter Carswell quoted in which Lawrence had written, in relation to the war, 'Children and child-bearing do not make spring. It is not in children the future lies ... There are many *enceinte* widows with a new crop of death in their wombs' (quoted p. 356). Wickham objects to this on two counts. First, like so many others, she objects to Lawrence's looseness of thought and language:

> He had no right to use the phrase '*enceinte* widows' symbolically, in some special sense, without giving a code to make his meaning clear. Lawrence does not attempt to put a meaning into words, he allows it to float on the breezes, odours, and free open spaces between his words. (pp. 356–7)

Secondly, she objects to Lawrence's denigration of female reproductive power:

> What possible sort of feeling could the passage I have quoted arouse but one of distrust of procreation ... Creation of hope is inferred to be male fertility, creation in life the silly yeasting of women ... Lawrence's irritable, ill-stated depreciation of procreation is the climax of his attack on women, the reduction *ad absurdum* of his hatred of them. (pp. 363–4)

As Wickham's critique suggests, in Lawrence's work pregnancy is assimilated to an increasingly idiosyncratic symbolic system, in which – as in the case of Ursula – female power/potency, especially in pregnancy, is experienced by men as deathly.

In the work of Katherine Mansfield, the symbolic or metaphorical significance of pregnancy is explored from a rather different angle. Through the perspective of her female characters, Mansfield challenges Freudian and Lawrentian readings of pregnancy as male gift and/or female appropriation of power. Mansfield's characters experience pregnancy as invasion and obliteration. In the short story 'Frau Brechenmacher Attends a Wedding' the motif of food suggests this understanding of pregnancy as compromising female autonomy. The comments of an anorectic patient, as given to the analyst Helmut Thoma, are pertinent here, confirming the metaphorical connections made by many women between food, sex and impregnation:

> Bottle – child – disgust, if I think of it – injections – the idea that there is something flowing into me, into my mouth or into the vagina, is maddening – integer, integra, integrum occurs to me – untouchable – he does not have to bear a child – a man is what he is – he does not receive and he does not give.[48]

In 'Frau Brechenmacher Attends a Wedding' food is everywhere: beer and sausages circulate among the guests, the bride's illegitimate daughter is force-fed to keep her quiet, the women have become fat and solid, hemming each other in. The bride is described as a cake ready to be cut into slices and served to others, but she is also taunted with the imminence of her own ingestion of food/impregnation:

> Herr Brechenmacher alone remained standing – he held in his hands a big silver coffee-pot. Everybody laughed at his speech, except the Frau; everybody roared at his grimaces, and at the way he carried the coffee-pot to the bridal pair, as if it were a baby he was holding.
>
> She lifted the lid, peeped in, then shut it down with a little scream and sat biting her lips. The bridegroom wrenched the pot away from her and drew forth a baby's bottle and two little cradles holding china dolls. As he dandled these treasures before Theresa the hot room seemed to heave and sway with laughter.[49]

Theresa's biting of her lips mirrors her daughter's attempts to refuse the sausages (she is a child who 'never did have a stomach'), and the image of force-feeding is linked with the rape-in-marriage which Frau Brechenmacher experiences and which will also be Theresa's lot. For such women, rape and pregnancy threaten both the integrity of the body and the wholeness of the self.

Mansfield's fullest treatment of pregnancy occurs in *Prelude* (1918), first drafted as the longer story *The Aloe* in 1915. In *Prelude* Linda Burnell is pregnant with her fourth child, the son who is born at the time of 'At the Bay', the second story of the 'Burnell' story-sequence. Linda's life has become a continuous 'prelude' because of her repeated pregnancies: like Anna Brangwen, she has become a 'threshold' for the life of others. She has become detached from everyday life and her husband, and experiences each of her pregnancies in terms of bodily assault:

> He was too strong for her; she had always hated things that rush at her, from a child. There were times when he was frightening – really frightening ... And at those times she had longed to say the most coarse, hateful things ... 'You know I'm very delicate. You know as well as I do that my heart is affected, and the doctor has told you I may die any moment. I have had three great lumps of children already ...[50]

Using the framework of a dream sequence, Mansfield offers a reading of pregnancy which gives Freud's Oedipal narrative a new twist. As one of the first fictional accounts of the psychology of pregnancy from a female perspective, the dream is worth quoting in full:

> 'How loud the birds are,' said Linda in her dream. She was walking with her father through a green paddock sprinkled with daisies. Suddenly he bent down and parted the grasses and showed her a tiny ball of fluff just at her feet. 'Oh, papa, the darling.' She made a cup of her hands and caught the tiny bird and stroked its head with her finger. It was quite tame. But a funny thing happened. As she stroked it began to swell, it ruffled and pouched, it grew bigger and bigger and its round eyes seemed to smile knowingly at her. Now her arms were hardly wide enough to hold it and she dropped it into her apron. It had become a baby with a big naked head and a gaping bird-mouth, opening and shutting. Her father broke into a loud clattering laugh and she woke to see Burnell standing by the windows rattling the Venetian blind up to the very top. (p. 51)

As in 'Frau Brechenmacher Attends a Wedding', pregnancy is presented in terms of unwanted swelling and engulfment. Mansfield exploits the mechanism of condensation described by Freud in *The Interpretation of Dreams*, so that the bird Linda dreams of simultaneously signifies the tumescent penis, the baby and the maternal body which must ruffle and 'pouch' as the baby grows. Linda experiences the baby as a malevolent and parasitic being, smiling 'knowingly' as it grows bigger and bigger. She does not, then, desire the penis-baby which Freud would see as a gift from the father-lover, and resists maternal femininity. She remains passionately attached to her mother, reflecting that 'there was something comforting in the sight of her that [she] felt she could never do without', but she does not wish to stand in her mother's place. As the dream reveals, she sees herself as having been trapped into marriage through collusion between her father and husband. Walking in a paradisal field with her father, she has been deceived by the fairy-tale picture of marriage which he offers her, a 'darling ... ball of fluff'. The reality of the voracious husband and of babies with 'big naked heads' appals her, and the dream encodes her sense of betrayal and entrapment. None the less, Linda knows that 'I shall go on having children and Stanley will go on making money'. In this brief sentence, Mansfield alludes unobtrusively to the wider social context of Linda's pregnancies. As an uneducated middle-class girl, Linda has taken up the only profession available to her. She has been exchanged between father and husband, and the unspoken understanding is that she will reproduce to match Stanley's production/making of money. Mansfield foregrounds, however, the fact that there is an element of choice here and the text thus points to the complex cross-currents at play in such negotiations. Linda may not enjoy her pregnancies, but she chooses to play her part in the marriage because it provides security not just for her, but for the mother whom she 'cannot do without' and for her unmarried sister. Mansfield does not construct Linda as a passive victim, but as one who has made accommodations and choices in a specific social and cultural context.

By the time *Prelude* was published in 1918 the circumstances of women's lives had changed significantly, however, in both England and New Zealand, where *Prelude* is set. The story thus offers a retrospective critique made possible in part by the greater freedom and opportunities available to women in the early twentieth century.

4
Mass Production

Eugenics and social class

In the 1920s and 1930s eugenic ideas were widely debated in Britain. This was, in the main, a period of optimism and intense speculation in relation to the transformative possibilities of science. Such possibilities were explored in numerous texts written for the 'intelligent layman' and published in relatively cheap format in the 'Today and Tomorrow' and the 'Thinker's Library' series. J.B.S. Haldane, Ronald Macfie and Garet Garrett were among those who wrote for a general readership about advances in biological science and the extension of man's knowledge and control over his own body.[1] The 'eugenic problematic' was an unavoidable issue for these writers, whose perspectives ranged from enthusiastic support to carefully qualified criticism.[2] As was the case before the First World War, eugenic thought also made its way into medico-social texts, which were now increasingly occupied with public health issues.

A major issue for eugenicists in Britain in the inter-war years remained that of class. The fear of differential breeding resurfaced, but now with a new twist, exemplified by Grantly Dick Read's observation in *Natural Childbirth* (1933) that women of 'the hospital classes' (those who could not afford to pay for private medical attendance) had easier pregnancies and labours than those of the upper and middle classes, and thus reproduced more effectively. In his *Revelation of Childbirth*, he went further, asking whether the poor should receive what he saw as preferential treatment: 'The home life and economic conditions of women of the poorer classes are investigated, and no effort is spared to make motherhood a joy and not a burden. You will have to ask yourselves whether the middle and upper classes, who pay for private attention, receive the same standard of care and attention as "hospital" folk.'[3]

One episode which demonstrates the extent to which eugenic thought had invaded popular consciousness is that of Sylvia Pankhurst's 'eugenic baby'. Pankhurst had been anxious to have a child after recovering from health problems which she attributed to the strain of her involvement with the suffrage campaign; her son Richard was born in 1927. However, her refusal to marry the child's father led to a final break with her mother, Emmeline, with whom her relationship had always been difficult. Patricia Romero, Sylvia's biographer, suggests that it was in order to hit back at her mother that Sylvia approached the 'scandal sheet' *News of the World* with the story of her baby.[4] The paper ran the story on the front page of the 8 April 1928 edition under the heading '"Eugenic" Baby Sensation. Sylvia Pankhurst's Amazing Confession', alongside a photograph of mother and child.

In her 'confession', which was syndicated round the world, Pankhurst explains her reasons for having a child using standard eugenic terminology: 'I wanted a baby, as every complete human being desires parenthood, to love him and cherish him, to see him grow and develop and to leave behind me a being who will, I hope, carry on the best that is in me and in my stock.' The article continues:

Miss Pankhurst then proceeded to discuss eugenics. 'You ask if my baby boy is eugenic,' she said. 'It is good eugenics, I believe, if one desires parenthood, to consider if one is of sufficient general intelligence, bodily health and strength, and freedom from hereditary diseases to produce AN INTELLIGENT AND HEALTHY CHILD [*sic*]. I believe that of myself. I believe that, also, of my baby's father. Indeed, I consider my 'husband' has many gifts with which to endow our child.[5]

The sensational element in this story lay principally in the fact that Pankhurst was an unmarried mother, and unapologetically so. It is difficult to assess to what extent her 'eugenic' claims would have been considered shocking by the paper's readers: the major point seized on in the article was that the father of the child was a 53-year-old 'foreigner' (Silvio Corio, an Italian, was in fact 52).

Prompted by her experiences of pregnancy, Pankhurst published a polemical book on motherhood, *Save the Mothers*, in 1930. Unlike Dick Read, she felt that only those who had access to private health care could be certain of receiving appropriate treatment. Accordingly, much of her book is taken up with arguments for increased state provision for maternity. Many of her proposals are far-sighted: they include not only a free maternity service but a £10 maternity bounty and payments for working mothers before and after the birth. None the less, as we might expect from her *News of the World* article, Pankhurst's book is inflected with the discourse of eugenics as well as that of social policy. Her main emphasis is on the benefits to be gained for mothers and the nation from public health initiatives. However, there is a counter-discourse which implies that, as well as saving mothers, the state might wish to prioritise those most fit to contribute to the nation's 'stock'. The patronising tone which Pankhurst adopts when describing 'puny babes' in 'dismal' tenements suggests that not many suitable contributions would come from the working class.[6]

As we saw in chapter 3, the class bias of British eugenic thought was bound up with the influence of the Eugenics Society, whose preoccupation in the 1930s was establishing a link between 'feeble-mindedness' and social class. The Society was particularly well represented on the committee that prepared the 1929 Wood Report on the incidence of mental deficiency in the population. This report came up with the definition of a 'social problem' group, which comprised 'the lowest 10% on the social scale': it was claimed that this group was associated not only with feeble-mindedness but also with insanity, epilepsy, pauperism, crime, unemployability and alcoholism.[7] The Society was also represented on the committee that produced the 1934 Brook Report on sterilisation, which endorsed the argument for voluntary sterilisation of those who could be classed as part of the social problem group. Following the Report, a Joint Committee on Voluntary Sterilisation was formed, which included representatives of the Central Association for Mental Welfare, the National Council for Mental Hygiene and the Eugenics Society. The Joint Committee campaigned widely between 1934 and 1940 and gained the support of the Royal Colleges of Physicians and Surgeons and the Royal College of Nursing. It is significant that about half the groups voting in support of voluntary sterilisation were women's organisations; these included the National Conference of Labour Women, the Conservative Women's Reform Association, the National Council of Women and about eighty women's co-operative guilds.[8]

Eugenic thought forms an important sub-text of Enid Bagnold's best-selling novel *The Squire*, which was published in 1938 and serialised in the same year in *Good Housekeeping* in Britain and the *Ladies Home Journal* in the US. Bagnold's novel is in some respects radical and pioneering in its detailed descriptions of pregnancy and childbirth, exploring, for example, the split subjectivity of the pregnant woman:

'The baby seemed to swim and strike like a dolphin. "It is a mystery," she said. "Women bearing children ... I shall become two people." ... She was a vase, a container, a split oak for a gnome to live in, a split oak, a hollow elm.'[9] Its account of labour is explicit, and follows the teachings of Grantly Dick Read, who argued that women should not resist contractions but should relax into them. In line with this advice, Bagnold writes: 'Now the first twisting spate of pain began. Swim then, swim with it for your life. If you resist, horror, and impediment! If you swim, not pain but sensation!' (p. 145). For some male readers this was too much. H.G. Wells protested in a letter to Bagnold that the book had made him feel that 'I'd been attacked by a multitude of many-breasted women (like Diana of Ephesus) and thrown into a washing basket full of used nursery napkins'.[10] However, the book undoubtedly fulfilled a useful function in providing information and reassurance at a time when many women, as doctors were quick to complain, still knew little about the processes of pregnancy and childbirth.

The novel is unabashed in its endorsement of class-based eugenics. Bagnold had long contemplated what she thought of as a book about motherhood: it turned out to be a book on eugenic motherhood. Her expectant mother (the 'squire' of the title, who is never named, but whose title suggests her powerful and controlling personality) heads a household based on a rigid social order, the rightness of which is never questioned. The only flaw in the regime which supports the squire's life is that hardy perennial in women's writing of the period, the 'servant problem'. The squire has difficulty in retaining domestic staff and becomes despondent whenever a staffing problem arises, particularly in the period covered by the novel when she is about to give birth. However, there is no consideration in the novel of the causes of the 'servant problem'. Rather, the squire expresses casual contempt for her servants, particularly the 'temporaries': 'They went from situation to situation with slovenly adaptability, shedding disruption about the house, Pied Piper whistling to its rats, a come-up-and-follow-me which got into the blood of the "unders," slackening discipline' (pp. 72–3). Servants are not only described metaphorically as animals (rats or birds), but are also associated with physical defects. An applicant for the post of cook peers 'over the pale trunk of an immense goitre', only to be characterised by the squire as 'a born lavatory attendant if ever there was one'; another servant girl is dismissed (literally and metaphorically) as a 'half-baked' and 'useless human being'. The implication is that, as a class, servants are defective and/or underdeveloped, and cannot be taught or helped.

Bagnold goes on to suggest that because the servant class is biologically inferior, it is unsuitable for reproduction. Significantly, none of the servants in the novel has children: they see their role, rather, as serving the fecund squire who is pregnant with her fifth child. Their own lives are entirely subsumed in her service, to the extent that the nursery governess is 'transfigured' by the news that labour is about to start, with 'happy excitement ... flying in her face'. The suggestion is that this is how things should be, with the sterile and 'half-baked' serving the strong and productive. The squire's fitness for reproduction is never in doubt. On the contrary, it is underscored through the midwife's thoughts as she approaches the squire's house:

> They were old hands, she and the squire. This was the fifth time they had worked together. She knew the squire had laid her ground well and was in fine condition, brown as a light loaf from head to foot, and strong ... She had no need in this case for her resolutions and her armour. The squire could be disciplined and good. (p. 112)

The reference to the midwife's 'armour' is noteworthy. Motherhood was frequently compared with military service in texts of this period, following the panic over the quality and quantity of the nation's stock in the context of war in Europe.[11] Bagnold's midwife is described elsewhere as 'a Religious and a crusador [sic]', engaged, so to speak, in a holy war for the production of healthy babies. In her conversations with the squire, she not only privileges some mothers over others but also advocates the establishment of maternity clinics, places of training for pregnant women to enable them to maximise their reproductive health and potential:

> My clinic would be a palisaded place, far in the country. There the mother should travel beforehand, passing through the isolation of a journey, leaving husband and family with their pre-occupations in the world. There, in a camp, like an athlete in training she should do her work for the newborn out of sight of life. No legends, no nonsense. The highest medical efficiency. Pre-natal observations carried out ... (p. 121, Bagnold's ellipsis)

In this utopian vision, which the squire endorses, once mothers had been selected and isolated, the foetus would be watched over and worked on. The reference to pre-natal observations recalls Ballantyne's idea of a 'pro-maternity hospital', but Bagnold's training camp has ideological overtones which would have appalled Ballantyne. The potential overlap between Bagnold's support for eugenics and support for Fascism was made explicit in November 1938 when she published an article in the *Sunday Times* praising 'Hitler's New Form of Democracy'. The article's calm acceptance of the transportation of the Jews shocked her friend, Violet Bonham Carter, who wrote to Bagnold that what surprised her most was that 'you could write with such irresponsible lightness, almost gaiety, of a situation undermined with human tragedy and horror'.[12]

Bagnold's novel offered a populist version of British eugenic thought, which had long focused on 'breeding out' the pauper class and social problem group. However, such a preoccupation could not survive the far-reaching ideological, structural and economic changes brought about by the Second World War. Thus, when in 1945 concerns about the falling birth rate were expressed (just as they had been after the Boer War and after the First World War), commentators took a different line from writers of earlier periods. In the inter-war years, medico-social writers had focused almost exclusively on the quality of the nation's stock and were preoccupied with the falling birth rate among the professional classes and with its 'dysgenic' consequences. After the Second World War, however, writers like G.F. McCleary, the author of several books on population issues, wrote optimistically about the possibilities of improving the health of all classes through environmental measures. In his *Race Suicide?* (1945), McCleary robustly attacked the older eugenicist 'lamentation about the falling birth-rate', which 'springs from the belief that wealthy people, regarded as transmitters of hereditary qualities, are superior in social value to poor people. Their wealth, it is alleged, is evidence of their superior intelligence. Similarly, according to this line of argument, poverty is a mark of inferior intelligence.' He writes of examples of genius arising in circumstances of poverty (he cites Schubert and Mozart) and questions the validity of IQ tests, pointing out the importance of upbringing and surroundings in enabling children to score well in such tests:

It is now generally accepted that environment plays an important part in the results of intelligence tests. This is a significant and encouraging conclusion; for a modern civilised community is already equipped to remove the unsatisfactory environmental conditions that bar the way to equality of opportunity for its poorer members. Methods of social amelioration have been worked out, and are being applied with increasing effect to raise the standards of life of the under-privileged.

For McCleary, the health and 'quality' of the nation could be improved by environmental health measures, while better state support for mothers offered the best means of encouraging a rise in the birth rate.[13]

In *Children for Britain*, also published in 1945, in a series which had Ernest Beveridge and Julian Huxley on the editorial board, Grace Leybourne-White and Kenneth White linked the decline in the birth rate with an increased desire for social mobility and with the spread of contraceptive knowledge (and aspirations) across class boundaries. They note that women were increasingly reluctant to have large families, quoting a telling letter from *The Labour Woman* of December 1943:

> The mothers of to-day have seen the conditions created by large families. They have seen their mothers toiling 16 hours a day, washing, scrubbing, cooking, nursing, and engaged in a constant struggle against poverty ... The effect of all these experiences has been a determination that this shall not be repeated in their own lives.[14]

Another factor was women's desire for 'a full life', which must somehow be reconciled with their 'unique function of motherhood'. A Commons statement by Dr Edith Summerskill is quoted in relation to this: 'There is another reason for the fall in the birth-rate ... Increasingly, women in this country want a career. We have a social system in which we compel women to choose between a career and motherhood' (p. 51).

Leybourne-White and White offer a balanced survey of the reasons for the continued decline in the birth rate and make practical suggestions for the support of families. Like McCleary they are in favour of children's allowances, and argue for more maternity beds and free nutrition for poorer pregnant women. They stress the importance of the environment, including the antenatal environment, in promoting a healthy race: 'every attention must be paid to the environment of all our children, from the moment of conception or before; for, if that is done, improvements in the child's qualities through "nurture" may well overcome inferior gifts of "nature"'. None the less, traces of the eugenics problematic remain in this study: the authors comment on the importance of the 'quality' of the race and on the need for those of 'higher than average powers of body or mind' to make the 'maximum contribution' to the population. And while in the post-Holocaust context they could hardly propose an explicitly eugenic solution to race anxieties, they do express concern about falling numbers among the population of the Dominions and raise the spectre of an increase in the 'the Asiatic multitudes' so great that 'parts of the Empire might be overwhelmed'. Moreover, this is not just an issue of numbers and power, but one of quality. The 'Anglo-Saxon character' of the Empire must be preserved, not diluted by 'the absorption of newcomers brought up in an alien culture'. The solution for Leybourne-White and White, then, is not immigration, but emigration:

> Emigration from Britain has been the cement of the Empire. If we wish to preserve Imperial unity, it must be done through the diffusion of people of British origin and culture. Hence, the more any shrinkage of numbers can be checked, the easier will be the solution of Imperial problems, and the surer will be our future as a first-class world power. (p. 42)

The 1949 Report of the Royal Commission on Population also raised concerns about the impact of the falling birth rate on the nation and the race. It was argued that it could impede industrial progress and might also compromise 'the development and cohesion of the Commonwealth' and the spread of British ideas, traditions and institutions throughout the world: 'the maintenance and extension of Western values, ideas and culture'.[15] Thus, while the class-based British eugenic project seems to have petered out at this point, the shadow of selective breeding persists in relation to the category of race. While commentators such as McCleary resist the notion of the 'fit' and 'unfit' as defined by social class, there is a more or less unexamined assumption in these texts that the Anglo-Saxon race must be protected (and perhaps promoted) because of its inherently superior quality.

The decline in the influence of class-based eugenics was due not only to the effects of the Second World War but to the development of alternative perspectives in genetic research. One of the most influential figures in this respect was J.B.S. Haldane, whose major scientific contribution was in uniting Darwinian evolutionary theory with Mendelian genetics.[16] Between 1924 and 1934 Haldane published a series of papers exploring genetic diversity and its relation to evolution. His conclusion, based on mathematical models, was that evolutionary change within a population takes place over a very long time-span. If this is the case, then eugenic sterilisation of so-called 'defectives' would have a minimal impact on a given population over any measurable period of time.[17] Haldane had been a member of the Labour Party in the 1920s, then moved further to the left in the 1930s, joining the Communist Party in 1942. He was a particularly effective critic of the eugenicists because of his scientific credentials, which enabled him to argue convincingly that, in its current state, genetics offered little certainty of improving the quality of the race. On the other hand, there was strong empirical evidence for the relatively rapid effectiveness of environmental interventions in improving the health of populations.

Ectogenesis

Haldane was one of the most successful early twentieth-century popularisers of science, a prolific journalist and radio commentator, who also produced books combining lucid exposition of scientific thought and speculation about future developments.[18] In *Daedalus*, which was published in 1924 and rapidly became a best-seller in Britain and the US, he explored the possibility of ectogenesis, that is, the production of a human being outside the body. He posits a technique whereby an ovary can be taken from a woman and kept growing 'in a suitable fluid for as long as twenty years, producing a fresh ovum each month, of which 90 per cent can be fertilised, and the embryos grown successfully for nine months, and then brought out into the air'.[19] In other words, he anticipates the development of the 'artificial womb'. Commenting on this development from the supposed perspective of a 'rather stupid undergraduate' of 2074, he writes that 'the effect on human psychology and social life of the separation of sexual love and reproduction ... is by no means wholly satisfactory'. However, the effects of selection outweigh these (unspecified) disadvantages, for 'the small proportion of men and women who are selected as ancestors for the next generation are so undoubtedly superior to the average that the advance in each generation in any single respect, from the increased output of first-class music to the decreased convictions for theft, is very startling' (p. 66). Haldane (unlike his 'rather stupid undergraduate') does not endorse selection, but anticipates it as a likely consequence if ectogenesis were to become possible. The suggestion in *Daedalus* is that human beings could be fertilised and grown in laboratory conditions in the foreseeable future (1951 is the date settled on) and Haldane is keen to alert his reader to the advantages and dangers attendant on such unprecedented control of the reproductive process.

Haldane's ambivalence about eugenics is reflected in his choice of title, for although the inventor Daedalus can be seen as a prototype modern scientific man, his gifts ultimately bring about the death of his son Icarus, who flies too close to the sun on wings Daedalus has made from feathers and wax.

Controlled reproduction is also the theme of Charlotte Haldane's speculative fiction *Man's World* (1926). The journalist Charlotte had contacted Haldane after reading an abridged version of *Daedalus*, hoping he would help her with her projected novel on the possibilities of sex-selection. At their first meeting in the summer of 1924 Haldane deluged her with information and with suggestions for further reading. He continued to advise and assist her, and they married in 1926.[20] *Man's World* was widely and favourably reviewed and constitutes a significant intervention in debates of the day about eugenics and ectogenesis. Rather like Huxley's *Brave New World*, it is a contradictory work which draws attention to the ambivalent possibilities of a society organised on 'scientific', rationalist lines. The society of Haldane's novel, Nucleus, is for the white 'race' only: other races live in different territories. Nucleus is organised for health, stability and control of the environment, and is strictly hierarchical, the mass of the people being controlled by a small (male) elite. Women can derive power only from 'vocational motherhood', a career for which only the finest specimens are selected: 'these mothers, radiant in the consciousness of their sublime mission to the race, were a group apart and uplifted'.[21] Haldane's main emphasis, however, is not on the selection of these mothers, but on the work they must carry out in pregnancy. They are trained in such topics as hygiene and childcare before they are mated (the passive voice seems appropriate here), and once pregnant are despatched to the kind of antenatal training camp envisaged in Bagnold's *The Squire*:

> Here they came, conscious of their chosen vocation, submitting willingly to the stringent discipline of hygiene, striving to attain physical and mental perfection, poise, and balance, and to transmit it to those born to the high wonder of scientifically directed living … Each mother knew in advance what would be the sex of the child to be born to her, and could aid its shaping to its destined end by judicious application under expert direction of the necessary mental and physical exercises. (p. 54)

Such training is necessary precisely because control of reproduction is not yet complete, although ectogenesis is on the horizon and is eagerly anticipated by male scientists such as Bruce Wayland in *Man's World*: 'Imagine it,' Bruce took up the completion of the thought, 'ectogenesis provides the means to select on the most strictly accurate lines. The numbers of mothers chosen diminish year by year. Until at last, those who supply the race are the supreme female types humanity can produce. Pyramidal' (pp. 61–2). Bruce's enthusiasm calls attention to a discrepancy: the principle of selection is not extended in the same way to men. There is no suggestion that the sperm, as opposed to the ovum, might eventually come from a few archetypal donors. It is surely significant that Bruce envisages variation as deriving from male sperm, while female input to reproduction would, ideally, be limited to a few selected breeders: this certainly seems to be a 'man's world' in terms of participation in and control of reproduction.

Only two characters offer any serious resistance to state-controlled reproduction. Encouraged by her brother, Nicolette attempts to take control of her fertility, refusing to mate with the young man who has been selected for her at the time when she has reached her reproductive peak. However, her rebellion is short-lived; as soon as she becomes pregnant by a man she prefers (the scientist Bruce, mentioned above) she lapses into the role she has been trained for:

> Already the embryo in her womb was to her Someone, was her son, and the sun that caressed her eyes, the perfumes which delighted her nose, the food she ate, the sleep which refreshed her, were His; passing to Him by the marvellous processes of which she knew a little. (p. 250)

The fate of her brother Christopher is more disturbing: disappointed in his sister and troubled by rebellious impulses and mystical longings, he commits suicide. His mysticism (which is thought aberrant and abnormal) is attributed to sexual indeterminacy, which is in turn attributed to his mother's failure to play her part in confirming the sex of her son. While pregnant with him she 'carried on all those exercises prescribed to develop the masculinity of the growing embryo listlessly. She was not disobedient but rather unobedient ... at a time when sex was still a matter more or less of experiment and the most stringent precautions were necessary in order successfully to coerce nature, it had its effect' (p. 86). Her son is incompletely masculine and therefore not fit for the purpose for which he has been bred, that of joining, and perpetuating, the governing elite. His 'self-ending' is presented as inevitable in a society which will not tolerate those who question or disrupt its progress. However, Christopher's resistance to the scientific rationalism of Nucleus is sympathetically presented, and his hostile conversations with Bruce bring into view the hidden ideological imperatives of his society. Nucleus rests on a definition of the human being as Aryan, exclusively heterosexual and, as far as possible, standardised. Christopher's mysticism, wayward individualism and sexual indeterminacy, while they set him apart from 'the army of propagatives', also make him something of a heroic outsider. Haldane's representation of his death as he flies his plane up to 'the forbidden heights' again invokes the myth of Icarus, whose death can be attributed in part to the hubris of his father.

The primary and unresolved tension in Haldane's novel is thus between scientific rationalism and romantic individualism, the principle of scientific rationalism being interrogated primarily in its relation to reproductive technology. And while *Man's World* cannot be represented as offering an unequivocal critique of scientific rationalism, the text does raise the question of whether science (or reason) can ever be value-free. Haldane's hesitation creates a novel which is simultaneously utopian and dystopian. Disease and physical suffering have been eliminated in Nucleus – but so have many human beings. Haldane underscores this last point in a passage which describes the reactions of the founder of this society to the (anticipated) Holocaust of the Second World War:

Most human life, of the quality then being cancelled, did not call to him for rescue. Human life – the cantmongers for centuries had been satisfied to extol its sanctity and to encourage its wasting and rotting by the slow disintegration of disease and death. The swifter process was the cleaner. Let the flames leap and lick, and the gases stifle and strangle. (p. 22)

In 1927 Haldane published a polemical text that has a more curious attitude to controlled reproduction. *Motherhood and Its Enemies* is explicit in its opposition to eugenics: in it Haldane warns that

this science holds potentialities of great danger. Let the class-conscious or race-proud individual with a capacity for stating sophistries with all the weight of learned argument, but with a mere smattering of scientific knowledge, attain any influence in this matter, and those whom he fears or hates (the same thing) will fare hardly.[22]

Yet she also contends that the 'enemies' of motherhood are primarily those women who are, in her words, 'sexually abnormal or sub-normal'. Quoting from a paper by Julian Huxley, she argues that such women belong 'if not to a "third sex", at least to a *third sexual category*' (p. 132; emphasis in the original). Appearing to conflate those who belong to this 'third sexual category' with the 'superfluous women' who outnumbered men in the inter-war period, she goes on to claim that 'intersexual' women have 'since the days of the suffragette, endeavoured to direct public opinion with regard to their sex' and that, in the years since the war, they have diverted attention from the 'exertions of mothers who had to carry, bear, and rear infants on insufficient rations or in other circumstances of considerable hardship'. She goes on:

> I believe that a conflict between the interests of these types and the interests of the mothers not only exists, but that owing to ignorance or propaganda it has so far been overlooked. In regarding these women as normals, and particularly in giving them political rights, modern society is encouraging them to put forward their pro-grammes as those of all womanhood, and I think we may easily find herein one reason for the present and progressive dislike for the home, 'womanly' occupations, and motherhood. (pp. 133–4)

It is difficult to reconcile this extraordinary attack on the 'third sex' with Haldane's anti-eugenic stance and with the sympathetic treat-ment of Christopher in *Man's World*. The explanation may lie in the fact that, as Jane Lewis and Susan Squier have argued, the ideology of motherhood was so prominent in this period that attachment to it offered the best – even the only – chance for feminists to further the case for women's rights.[23] Thus it could be argued that in *Motherhood and Its Enemies* Haldane promotes the ideal of vocational motherhood because she is aware that this is one of the best cards that women can play in a society that cannot yet manage to reproduce itself without the bodies of women. And the case for valuing and supporting the ideal mother can best be made by contrasting her with 'abnormal' women, who pose a threat to all social norms – according to Haldane, their 'fanaticism and crankiness have caused them to take up freak science, freak religions, and freak philanthropy' (p. 155).

Such an interpretation can be supported if we read *Motherhood and Its Enemies* alongside Aldous Huxley's *Brave New World*, by far the best-known fantasy about reproductive technology. In *Brave New World* things have gone further than in *Man's World*: ectogenesis is now a fact and complete control of the reproductive process is possible. In this capitalist utopia/dystopia, individuals have been replaced by social units, bred and conditioned to play their part in production and (more importantly) consumption. Although, as David Bradshaw has pointed out, Huxley was flirting with the possibilities of eugenics around the time of the novel's publication, his numerous essays come out, on balance, against eugenics and controlled reproduction; as he suggests in his 1927 'A Note on Eugenics', human beings are not sufficiently well informed to be able to 'improve' the race.[24] *Brave New World* does not, however, offer an unequivocal critique of controlled reproduction and/or reproductive technology. For example, Huxley's account of the laboratory where the 'babies in bottles' are bred endows an apparently soul-less technological process with seductive warmth and colour: he describes the scene of artificial reproduction in terms of a 'sultry darkness ... visible and crimson, like the darkness of closed eyes on a summer afternoon', in which the rows of bottles 'glinted with innumerable rubies'.[25] In contrast, viviparous reproduction is associated with the hideous Linda, the biological mother of the Savage and a bloated, sagging, middle-aged alcoholic. Biological motherhood is also linked with monstrous femininity in the world-controller's description of family life in the past: 'Maniacally, the mother brooded over her children (*her* children) ... "My baby, and oh, oh, at my breast, the little hands, the hunger, and that unspeakable agonizing pleasure!"'(p. 33). Although this can be read as an ironic commentary on the misguided values of the 'brave new world', a sense of disgust in relation to 'natural' pregnancy is none the less powerfully expressed. In its response to the elimination of pregnancy and its replacement by *in vitro* fertilisation/gestation, the text thus seems more than a little in love with the technological advances it is often believed to condemn.

Moreover, in *Brave New World* all the positions of power and social control are held by men: the women are reduced to essentially menial functions (tending embryos in bottles and babies in nurseries). One can infer from this that once reproduction has been separated not just from sex, but from women's bodies, women as a social group lose an important means to power – however indirect and derivative such power might be. Without the bargaining tool of what Haldane called 'vocational motherhood', they have no means of access to or input into the decision-making process. It is sobering to reflect that in the context of British society in the 1930s, such a situation seemed to Huxley the logical outcome of the developments he imagined and anticipated. In this context ectogenesis, far from promising to free women from biological servitude (as later feminists were to contend) could be viewed as constituting a serious threat to their social and political position.

The debates over controlled reproduction of the 1920s and 1930s must be set in the context not only of scientific advances and debates about motherhood, but in a wider political context. This was a period of economic and social instability throughout Europe. In Britain the depression brought mass unemployment, and the economic crisis of 1931 forced the formation of the first National Government. For intellectuals such as the Haldanes and the Huxleys, Soviet Russia, with its centralist government and five-year economic plans, seemed to offer a more viable model than Britain or the US for the creation of a stable, egalitarian society.[26] The USSR was also a society in which reproduction, as well as production, was considered a social rather than an individual matter, a legitimate area for state intervention. This development found an echo in the contemporary movement towards a national maternity policy in Britain.

The national

The development of a national framework of antenatal care in Britain falls into two stages, pre- and post-National Health Service. The pattern of provision in the 1920s and 1930s was uncoordinated, to say the least. Maternity care was provided by local authorities via clinics and health visitors, and by municipal and voluntary hospitals, which offered clinics and beds for confinement. Midwives, municipal clinic medical officers, GPs and hospital obstetricians offered a range of services, but were often responsible to different authorities, and there was no provision for passing on information about individual cases. It was widely agreed that universal – and standardised – antenatal care should be available, involving at least three visits, with an initial pelvic examination followed by routine monitoring of blood pressure and urine analysis.

Women proved unexpectedly resistant to the idea, however. In the 1927 edition of *The Queen Charlotte's Practice of Obstetrics* it is noted that the fact that medical supervision is necessary throughout pregnancy is 'hardly realised even at the present time'. The authors optimistically claim that most of the difficulties of pregnancy, notably the high maternal death rate from haemorrhage, eclampsia and the complications of labour, would be eliminated if 'preventive obstetrics' were better developed. Thus: 'Once a woman has engaged her medical attendant it should be made clear to her that his advice is always to be obtained.'[27] This hortatory tone seems to have been common: in a 1933 booklet based on a series of radio talks for pregnant women, Eardley Holland writes that as antenatal clinics are widely available there is 'no excuse' for an expectant mother not to have antenatal care: 'But, and I must emphasize this very strongly, there is reason to believe that a very large number of women, even at the present time, do not avail themselves of it. This must be due either *to ignorance or to slack-ness*. Be sure that you receive ante-natal care, and teach your friends and acquaintances to do likewise.'[28]

The motives behind the drive to persuade women to attend for ante-natal screening were complex. Ann Oakley has linked this drive with a desire for professional dominance and with the profession's 'attempt to control the behaviour of women's bodies'.[29] She has also suggested that the professional 'commandment' that women should attend for ante-natal care was enforced all the more vigorously as women became enfranchised and threatened to act with greater independence. Yet one could turn this argument round and argue that it was women them-selves who demanded better antenatal care as they gained access to the public sphere. The most influential campaigners for antenatal care were after all not obstetricians but women like the health campaigner Margery Spring Rice, who worked with the medical profession to secure the information and services women were asking for. It was Spring Rice who argued forcefully that antenatal care should include basic educa-tion about the physiology of pregnancy and the mechanisms of labour, as well as screening for conditions such as pre-eclampsia: the need for such information had been stressed repeatedly by the contributors to Margaret Llewelyn Davies' *Maternity*.

Many obstetricians were also aware of the social and gender implica-tions of antenatal care and of the ways in which women could be failed by an impersonal system. For example, in the first edition of F.J. Browne's *Antenatal and Postnatal Care*, which ran to nine editions between 1935 and 1960, the author noted that maternal mortality had not fallen despite Ballantyne's optimism expressed twenty years earlier, and that the death rate from eclampsia has also changed little. He concluded that this was due to the current inadequacy of antenatal care, an inadequacy which, significantly, he defines in terms of the lack of a good relationship between doctor and patient: 'Much of that which now passes under the guise of antenatal care is unworthy of the name. Examinations are too infrequent, too perfunctory and too unskilled to accomplish anything useful.' He goes on to insist that patients must be individualised, and writes that in the antenatal clinic *'there should be no such thing as mass production'*.[30]

Browne's explicit use of a metaphor drawn from industrial production is striking. It offers a critique of the relations between obstetricians and patients anticipating by decades that of feminist critics such as Barbara Rothman, who argued in 1989 that reproduction had become a form of alienated labour: 'As babies and children become products, mothers become producers, pregnant women the unskilled workers on a reproductive assembly line.'[31]

It seems that a lack of understanding of class, not of gender, was the major shortcoming of inter-war antenatal care: Margery Spring Rice's study *Working-Class Wives* seems to confirm this. As in *Maternity* and *A School for Mothers*, this study emphasises the sacrifices mothers make for their children, born and unborn, and their extreme reluctance to seek any medical assistance for themselves. In relation to this, the report notes a 'curious phenomenon': although more than 70 per cent of the women surveyed *consult* a doctor in illness, only about 5 per cent speak of having received any *health teaching* from a doctor. Conversely, although only 8 per cent *consult* antenatal or other welfare centres, 47 per cent speak of having *learnt about health* from such centres. Spring Rice infers from this that, in general, 'the mother is a great deal more careful and anxious to learn about the health of the children than about her own', and that when she visits a clinic she is often not conscious of having consulted them about herself, so that 'advice given to her for herself is incidental and often unsought'.[32] In other words, the question of the mother's health is best approached indirectly. However, the reasons for the mother's reluctance to seek help are in general those of brute economics, as a letter from a district nurse makes clear:

> It is mother who gets left out so far as treatment goes. She can go to hospital for teeth and so on but she cannot afford transport nor as a rule the time, and no-one pays for transport for her, unless she is so ill as to need to go into the hospital as an in-patient. She *may* get the 'family' doctor for herself as well as the children if she pays into the medical club ... If she does not pay in, she carries on as long as she possibly can without advice or treatment ... She will not start a doctor's bill for herself if she can possibly stand on her feet. (quoted pp. 66–7)

Thus, the failure of many women to take full advantage of antenatal care was not due to 'slackness' as Eardley Holland claimed, but to the wish to avoid all unnecessary costs: a visit to the antenatal clinic could result in advice being received, which, if acted on, would impact adversely on other members of the family.

In reality, the majority of problems occurring in antenatal health in this period were related primarily to social rather than to clinical factors. This became clear during and after the Second World War, which was, in the memorable words of Ann Oakley, 'the best thing that had happened to pregnant women for a long time'.[33] As she points out in her definitive account of the move from 'warfare to welfare', with fathers at war and mothers at work, families could no longer be considered self-sufficient, and the government had to step in to provide community care in the widest sense. In July 1940 a national milk scheme was introduced, providing a cheap pint daily for all expectant and nursing mothers, and in 1941 a vitamin welfare scheme was instituted. Expectant mothers and children under five also received an additional egg ration. At the end of the war the Ministry of Health could claim, with some justification, that these measures were the prime cause of a marked decline in maternal, neonatal, infant mortality and stillbirth rates.[34]

In addition to such nutritional measures, which continued after the war, the state also provided, in theory, a national maternity service from the date when the NHS Act came into force in 1948.[35] In practice, however, the service remained chaotic and uncoordinated. As before, the care of pregnant women could come from three different bodies: hospital authorities, GPs and local authorities. Communication between these authorities remained poor. By the end of the 1950s local authority clinics, previously the only source of free antenatal care, had declined in popularity, thus simplifying matters to some extent, as most women now received care from a combination of the GP and hospital antenatal clinic. However, there was no agreed strategy for antenatal care, and territorial struggles between GPs, midwives and hospital obstetricians created the potential for further confusion.

It could be argued that in the immediate post-war period, which was one of increased welfare provision and a generally higher standard of living, some of the more pressing problems of antenatal care had been mitigated. However, the problem noted by Browne of 'mass production' in antenatal care had, if anything, intensified. Thus in a survey published in 1948 under the auspices of the Royal College of Obstetricians and Gynaecologists and the Population Investigation Committee, it was reported that antenatal clinics were often held in unsuitable premises, divided into rooms by portable screens only.

Patients frequently had a hurried examination: invoking the spectre of antenatal 'time-and-motion' study, the survey describes one encounter which took just three minutes. The record of this consultation also reveals a division of labour between health visitor and consultant, a failure to attend to the individual patient's history and, more broadly, the reduction of the patient to a medical case:

> A health visitor interviewed the expectant mother outside the consultation room and recorded details of her history and present symptoms. The woman then removed her stockings and knickers behind a screen and, otherwise fully clothed, entered the consultation room ... Here she lay on a couch, her dress was pulled up, and her abdomen hurriedly palpated. The doctor listened to the foetal heart and asked two or three questions about a minor symptom of which she was complaining. No further examination was made and the doctor took no detailed history.[36]

In her account of having her first baby on the NHS, *National Baby*, Sarah Campion comments on the speed with which samples were taken, with nurses too busy even to speak, and reports an even more rapid examination by a doctor ($2\frac{1}{2}$ minutes). She disliked, too, the lack of privacy and objectification of her as a patient: 'I hated being pulled about and prodded; I hated sitting on hard public bunks in nothing but a brassiere and pants while all the world surged by: I hated having my body made the arena for a medical free-for-all.'[37] None the less, Campion's assessment was on the whole positive. She recognised the problem of reconciling the 'impersonal beneficence' of a mass system with the need to give mothers 'individual self-confidence', but concluded: 'in my experience, the ante-natal clinic came nearer to solving [the problem] than the hospital proper ... When we had been attending the clinic for half a year or more, we knew what we were about ... the clinic had taught us to trust ourselves' (pp. 149–50). Campion's account is also revealing about the class politics of NHS attendance in this period. Her sympathy with a tearful fellow patient is abruptly withdrawn when the woman 'confesses the worst grievance of all, which is the sudden leap in the price of privacy ... she, of course, must have a private room' (p. 14). Campion recognises that many middle-class women will continue to pay for private care, partly out of a desire for privacy, partly out of snobbery, but ends her book with an appeal to women of all classes to use the NHS. Her fear is that if middle-class women do not sign up to the NHS, it will not survive.

A.S. Byatt's novel *Still Life* (1985) offers a more critical view of ante-natal care during the 1950s. The chapter 'Ante-Natal: December 1953' draws attention to the phenomenon of 'block bookings' (twelve or more women booked for one appointment), the ensuing long waits and the general lack of dignity and privacy for pregnant women. The novel also highlights the repressive nature of the institution, the logic of which tends to become its own smooth running rather than the welfare of the individuals for whom it caters. In Byatt's fictional clinic, the bullying sisters and distant, overstretched doctors create a climate of helplessness and passivity which prove fatal: a patient loses her baby because, although she is haemorrhaging, she is too intimidated to demand attention. Stephanie Potter (one of the novel's central charac-ters) feels guilty because she hasn't listened to the woman's complaints when they were standing together in the queue. As she explains to the doctor, she too has learnt to be quiescent: 'This place puts you in line. You stay in it. You stand for *hours*, without a girdle, because of block bookings and not enough chairs ... This place changes you. I told her myself not to think.'[38] This takes us back to Browne's point about the dangers of 'mass production' and the issue of what Norman Morris was to call 'human relations in obstetric practice'. A recurring theme in writings on antenatal care over the centuries is the need to establish trust between doctor and patient: as, William Hunter himself had pointed out: 'It is not the mere safe delivery of the woman will recom-mend an accoucheur, but a sagacious well-conducted behaviour of tenderness, assiduity and delicacy.'[39]

The question of trust is critical because antenatal care is an anom-alous branch of medical practice: the 'patients' are not in the main ill, but want information and some degree of reassurance. Yet there is a structural problem in that the need for advice can draw the medical practitioner into areas such as emotional support in which s/he may have no expertise and into areas where s/he has no power – s/he cannot ensure that a woman receives adequate nutrition and rest. Byatt makes this point through her character's reflections on her doctor's well-meant platitudes. He urges her: 'Do stop crying. It does no good. Pregnancy is an upsetting time for some people. You must try and keep calm for your child's sake.' Stephanie 'did not feel angry with him: she could imagine how it was for him: woman after woman after woman, all the same, all different, weeping on occasion for fear, boredom, pain, frustration, humiliation. How could he take on all that, much of it irremediable, at ten-minute intervals?' (p. 16).

The question of mass production and its ill-effects was aired, as noted above, by Norman Morris in 'Human Relations in Obstetric Practice'. The article was based on a lecture given at the opening of a new obstetric unit at Charing Cross Hospital and drew on letters sent to a woman's magazine for evidence of women's feelings about ante-natal care. Many of the letters used metaphors drawn from factory production (for example, the conveyor belt) to describe the clinic expe-rience, and many drew attention to the instrumental way in which women were treated. Foucault's dictum that 'if one wishes to know the illness from which he is suffering, one must subtract the individual, with his particular qualities' is given an obstetric twist in the following anecdote:

> The nurses and doctors were very friendly at the antenatal clinic and very helpful – but – we were rather like 'sausages in a sausage machine'. I understood that there were far too many pregnant women and far too few doctors. It was rather amusing to hear the remark of a nurse on seeing one mother-to-be making her face up. She was told 'Don't bother with your face, dear, it's the other end he's interested in'.[40]

Morris argued for a refiguring of the relationship between doctor and patient based on a recognition of the patient as a fellow human being. He stressed that 'the mother-to-be is extremely vulnerable' and, return-ing to the question of trust, emphasised 'the importance of *words* and their impact on the patient' and the 'extraordinary value of kindness' in the relationship between doctor and patient. Such a perspective offered a challenge to the normative model of health care which had, as Christopher Lawrence notes, become 'almost incontestable' by the mid-twentieth century. This rested on a view of medicine as an encounter between doctor and illness rather than between doctor and patient. Because illness was defined as a pathology not particular to the individual, it was taken for granted that the treatment of the pathology (or, in the case of antenatal care, the search for the symptom) required little attention to individual emotional needs.[41]

The clinical usefulness of antenatal care was carefully evaluated in two articles published in 1960 in *The Lancet*, by Sir Dugald Baird, Regius Professor of Midwifery and Gynaecology at Aberdeen. Surveying forty years of obstetrics, Baird notes that by far the most important development in relation to maternal mortality has been the virtual elimination of puerperal sepsis. In relation to foetal mortality, Baird notes that the stillbirth rate remains higher in England and Wales than in many other countries, and also that it has not improved in the ten or more years since the introduction of the NHS. Analysing variations in stillbirth rates over the previous 30 years, he suggests a correlation between high unemployment in the late 1920s and early 1930s and a high stillbirth rate. Conversely, the fall in unemployment after 1933 can be linked to a fall in the stillbirth rate, which was further accelerated by the 'enlightened food policy' of the war years. In other words, foetal health is largely dependent on social and environmental factors, which have long-term, trans-generational effects. Thus, the health of a foetus depends not only on a good diet during pregnancy, but on the mother's general health and physique. These will be related, in turn, to factors in the mother's own childhood, including her diet. Thus in terms of the mother's effect on the foetus Baird argues that 'the diet consumed from birth to maturity is at least as important as the diet taken during pregnancy'.[42]

Looking at perinatal mortality rates – that is, the number of stillbirths and deaths in the first week of life per 1,000 births – Baird concludes that to reduce the rate much below the current level of just above 30 per 1,000 would require 'a considerable improvement in the general level of health and physique'. He argues that more research is needed into prematurity, which has replaced birth trauma as the major cause of perinatal mortality. He notes that 'although the management of the liveborn premature has improved, we know little about the reasons why foetal growth is impaired or why labour starts, whether it be at term or very much earlier'.[43] In other words, the *causes* of miscarriage, premature labour and growth retardation were not understood; nor, more importantly, was it possible to assess what was then termed 'placental insufficiency'. In these circumstances, the project of universal antenatal monitoring was beginning to seem somewhat irrelevant, as it could not anticipate the major causes of perinatal mortality. Baird does not say this explicitly, and it would be another twenty years before the *Lancet* would publish an article asking 'Is Routine Antenatal Care Worth While?', but the implication is there.[44] It is also significant that in considering the management of placental insufficiency among older multigravidae (women who had had multiple births – a high-risk group), Baird opts for a high-tech, interventionist route: 'Our investigations suggested that there is much to be said for induction of labour to avoid the risk of placental insufficiency ... and for a more liberal use of caesarean section to avoid undue stress to the baby in labour'.

The 'technologisation' of pregnancy can be said to have begun with the development of the first reliable pregnancy test in the 1920s. The Aschheim and Zondek (A–Z) test was based on the observation that the urine of pregnant woman contained higher than usual levels of oestrogen. It involved the use of animals to test such levels, initially only in cases where it was considered particularly important to establish a diagnosis. A 'Pregnancy Diagnosis Station' was set up in 1929 to take nationwide samples, and in its 1930 report describes a typical referral in these terms: 'patient very neurotic and convinced she is pregnant' (this turned out not to be the case). As the test became more sophisticated and less expensive, it was adopted as a matter of routine. Thus in place of 'touching' or physical examination by doctor or midwife, pregnancy was now diagnosed remotely, by sending a urine sample to a laboratory, and the result of the test was usually given by telephone. In her novel *The Virgin in the Garden*, Byatt dramatises such a telephonic annunciation in the surroundings of a public box smelling of 'stale tobacco, evaporated urine, warmed metal'.[45] Byatt here draws attention to the ways in which knowledge of pregnancy was being transformed by new technologies and procedures, becoming at once more reliable and more impersonal. This was to change once again with the development of home pregnancy testing kits, which brought reliability *and* privacy.

A further significant (and somewhat unfortunate) development was the adoption of X-ray techniques in order to diagnose pregnancy and determine gestational age. It is difficult to determine how widely X-rays were used for routine diagnosis: certainly in some areas in the 1920s and 1930s all pregnant women were referred for radiology. Although concerns were expressed about its safety, the practice continued during the 1940s and 1950s: at Queen Charlotte's Hospital the number of X-ray examinations as a proportion of patients delivered rose from 28.5 per cent in 1946 to 66.7 per cent in 1954.[46] In 1956, however, Alice Stewart published a study which implicated antenatal X-rays in the development of childhood cancer and this led to an immediate and rapid reduction in their use for diagnostic purposes. In any case, by the late 1950s a more sophisticated technique was being developed which would enable clinicians to monitor intra-uterine life. Ian Donald, Professor of Midwifery at Glasgow, drew on his knowledge of the naval echo-sounding technique of sonar to create ultrasound technology, publishing his first paper on the subject in the *Lancet* in 1958. The principle on which sonar was based was that when subjected to an electric charge, certain crystals emit high-frequency sound-waves which travel though water, sending back echoes when they encounter a solid object. Donald realised that a more sophisticated version of this technique could be used to detect and image foetal development. The introduction of ultrasound to obstetrics was a gradual process, however. Donald's 'contact B' scanner was used in the 1960s by enthusiastic obstetricians to detect placenta praevia, foetal growth retardation, and so on, but, as Stuart Campbell, Professor of Obstetrics and Gynaecology at King's College Hospital puts it, 'the dedication, experience and expertise required to use the heavy, unwieldy equipment was a scarce commodity. Ultrasound scanning during this period was generally regarded as a kind of art form which was nice to have if the local expertise was available.' The development of the real-time scanner was the 'desperately needed breakthrough' which brought cheaper, lighter and smaller equipment and which made scanning technically much easier.[47] As a result, by the late 1970s ultrasound had become the most common method of monitoring foetal development in the UK.

Enthusiasts such as Campbell hailed the introduction of ultrasound in obstetrics as 'one of the great revolutionary milestones' in the specialism. He added:

> A final, perhaps unexpected, benefit of the real-time revolution was that parents on seeing their fetus moving on the screen were informed and delighted and indeed the ultrasound session became a family event. Maternal–fetal bonding was accelerated … there was no doubt that parental acceptance of this particular form of high technology was reassuringly high. (pp. 369–70)

No evidence is given to support this bold assertion and, as we shall see in chapter 5, women's responses to ultrasound images vary widely, depending on social differences such as class and race, on biological differences such as age and fertility history, and on the medico-clinical context in which the scan takes place. The meaning of the ultrasound image cannot be assumed: it depends on the context in which it is received and interpreted.

The natural

The natural childbirth movement derived much of its impetus from a reaction against both 'mass production' and increasing technological intervention in obstetrics. As we have seen, many mothers were dismayed by the conveyer-belt approach to antenatal care, which they felt undermined rather than developed their self-confidence. Many also distrusted the medical profession's enthusiasm for technological developments: for example, a woman who was X-rayed in order to diagnose a twin pregnancy in the 1950s later confessed, 'I was a bit worried about having an X-ray when I was pregnant, but at that time you didn't feel you could question things. They were the professionals and they knew – you just took their word for it.'[48] The natural childbirth movement attempted to address the related issues of women's lack of self-confidence and the increased medicalisation of pregnancy and childbirth. It began with the work of Grantly Dick Read, who had become convinced that women experienced pain in childbirth because they anticipated pain. Fear caused their muscles to tense and the cervix to contract, making it difficult for the child to descend through the pelvis: 'fear of itself produces pain, and pain, terror, and so the agony of childbirth.'[49] The remedy was an approach to pregnancy and childbirth in which the patient had a good personal relationship with her doctor or midwife, was informed and supported throughout, and was taught relaxation and breathing exercises to help her in labour. Read's main focus was on the feelings of the prospective mother; he argued for the need to attend to these from the moment when the first arrangements for confinement were made:

> We overlook, perhaps, the excitement which attends these preliminary arrangements ... During pregnancy, the average girl needs considerable support; she requires explanation of unfamiliar occurrences ... The nurse and the doctor and the ante-natal clinic are responsible for her attitude towards childbirth.[50]

He also attacked the instrumental approach of many obstetricians to their patients, arguing that the emphasis of antenatal care was too often purely scientific, with physicians attending to 'the efficiency of machinery and metabolism' but failing to 'delve into the thoughts of women who appeal to them for help'. Pithily, he pointed out that in obstetrics, 'there is usually a woman present as well as a reproductory apparatus'.[51]

Read's arguments for what we would now call more holistic care were timely and compelling, although they were founded on some curious and unproven assumptions about the health of 'primitive' peoples and the poor. Thus in pregnancy he claimed:

> the primitive woman continues her work – in the harvest field, on trek, in the rubber plantation, or wherever she may be employed.

The child develops while she herself lives a full and natural existence. Muscularly strong, physiologically efficient, her mechanism carries out its normal functions without discomfort, difficulty or shame. The child then is born – small, hard and easily.[52]

He goes on to describe a birth he witnessed under 'a sub-tropical sun' which was so easy that he looked on, smoking his pipe throughout. This passage is typical of Read in its confident assertion on the basis of a single case about which he gives no circumstantial detail. His category of the 'primitive' is especially worrying in that it encompasses the ancient civilisations of China, India and Japan. His observations about 'the poor' may be based on a more tenable system of classification, but similarly lack supporting evidence. Read's thesis is that the poor are more in touch with 'reality' and natural process – that they are, in fact, more primitive. Hence their success in pregnancy and childbirth, for 'where life itself has entailed hardship and struggle for survival in society where the primitive instincts are not curbed, in environments which educate to a personal fortitude, fundamental experience does not come as an entirely new and unsuspected state to the young mother'.[53]

Read's work had an immediate impact, and his approach to pregnancy and childbirth was welcomed by many British obstetricians. F.J. Browne, for example, invited him to contribute a chapter on 'The Influence of the Emotions upon Pregnancy and Parturition' for the first edition of his *Antenatal and Postnatal Care*. Indeed, Read's approach fitted in with a long-standing tradition of conservatism and cautious intervention in British obstetrics, which can be traced from Thomas Denman's 1788 *An Introduction to the Practice of Midwifery* to successive editions of the influential *Queen Charlotte's Textbook of Obstetrics* in the twentieth century.[54] Read's philosophy could indeed more accurately be described as conservative rather than 'natural'. It was informed by contemporary scientific thought, drawing on a range of sources which included the work of the physiologist Sir Charles Sherrington on the role of nociceptors in the perception of pain, and it did not rule out the use of analgesia.

'Nature' and 'the natural' are in any case extraordinarily mobile concepts/constructions – as witness the fact that the most influential contemporary scientific journal is called *Nature*. In using the term 'natural', Read certainly intended to suggest a non-interventionist approach and to call up the post-romantic connotations of nature as a benevolent, even mystical force. For Read, pregnancy was a spiritual, even religious experience. In *Revelation of Childbirth* he contends that pregnancy,

> free from anxiety and fear, is characterised by a profound urge for a fuller and more lucid knowledge of the spiritual forces of life. Women have spoken of an incomprehensible elation, a sense of inner rejoicing, that sweeps them away from mundane realities to new worlds in which for days on end they live a life of physical and mental exaltation. Mere man is rarely sensible of the irresistible emotional transformation that underlies natural pregnancy. (pp. 137–8)

Read may have been drawing here on Bagnold's poetic evocation of pregnancy in *The Squire*. It is likely that Bagnold had read *Natural Childbirth*, and Read may have returned the compliment when Bagnold's novel was published in 1938. Bagnold describes pregnancy in terms of 'exaltation' and also points to the experience within it of a new relation to time. She writes,

> a child in the womb or at the breast stops time. Time stands still. Death recedes ... Half-dazed, half-mystic, she had felt the walls of her life stretch and grow thin ... had wandered about the house, touching her children, talking to them, released from life, released from time, released from death. She had then no need to be quick before eternity. (p. 153)

For Bagnold, as 'the walls of her life' grow thin, the pregnant woman is released from time and mortality and at the same time moves closer to what lies beyond life and death. Her perspective overlaps with Julia Kristeva's account of 'maternal' female subjectivity. In 'Women's Time' Kristeva argues that such subjectivity is associated with cyclical time ('the eternal return of biological rhythm that is similar to the rhythm of nature') and monumental time ('all-encompassing and infinite, like imaginary space'). Kristeva is careful to point out that 'repetition and eternity serve as fundamental conceptions of time in numerous experiences, notably mystical ones' and that this relationship to time is not incompatible with masculine subjectivity. None the less, in this and other essays, she insists on the possibility of pregnancy as a state of grace, as part of her critique of Christian representations of maternity.[55]

Doris Lessing broke many taboos in the representation of female bodily experience and, in her preface to the second edition of *The Golden Notebook* (1963), commented wryly on the stir caused by her references to menstruation in that novel. In *A Proper Marriage*, published two years later, she took on the representation of pregnancy, possibly an even more 'improper' subject for a novelist. Like Bagnold, Lessing suggests that pregnancy is accompanied by temporal dislocations and suggests too that these shifts in temporal perspective bring a fuller understanding of the forces involved in human development. Through the consciousness of Martha Quest (the central character in the novel-sequence *Children of Violence*), Lessing presents the experience of pregnancy in terms which echo Freud's argument that ontogeny recapitulates phylogeny.[56] Extending the frame of reference within which pregnancy is interpreted, Lessing links pregnancy imaginatively with conceptions of pre-history, as she stretches the concept of ontogeny to include pre-natal life:

> The moment Douglas had gone to the office, Martha drifted to the divan, where she sat, with listening hands, so extraordinarily compelling was the presence of the stranger in her flesh. Excitement raced through her; urgency to hurry was on her. Yet, after a few minutes, these emotions sank. She had understood that time, once again, was going to play tricks with her. At the end of the day, when Douglas returned from the office, she roused herself with difficulty, dazed. To her it was as if vast stretches of time had passed. Inside her stomach the human race had fought and raised its way through another million years of its history; that other time was claiming her.[57]

Pursuing the theme of the pre-historical and pre-cultural, Lessing subsequently depicts the naked, pregnant Martha wallowing in the mud (the primeval slime), her child protected from the elements only by 'half an inch of flesh'.

While there is no evidence to suggest that Lessing had read Dick Read, her fictional accounts of pregnancy accord with his ideals and in her autobiography she presents her own pregnancies in terms of healthy nature triumphing over medical rules and constraints. She also powerfully conveys the sense of hostility between pregnant women and the medical establishment which was developing in the 1950s and 1960s. The struggle as she presents it was a reworking of the eighteenth-century debate between Nihell and Smollett, discussed in chapter 1. Who had the right to speak of pregnancy? And how was it best known – through the pregnant woman's perceptions or the medical practitioner's gaze? Lessing explains:

> In those days, you did not dare say your baby had 'quickened' long before the official three and a half months, and that when still in the womb the creature responded to your thoughts and your

moods. No use saying that your infant knew your voice from birth
... To such claims the doctors would say patronizingly you were
imagining it, women did imagine things.[58]

Although Lessing's experience was in Southern Rhodesia, this gender-
inflected debate was also intensifying in Britain and the US. It was in part
a side-effect of Read's work and was stimulated in Britain by the Natural
Childbirth Association, of which he was the first president. The
Association had been founded in 1956 by Prunella Briance, whose second
child had died following conventional obstetric care. She was convinced
that the death would have been averted if Read's non-interventionist
approach to labour had been followed, and was intent on making his
work more widely known. In this she was extremely successful: the
launch of the Natural Childbirth Association in 1957 attracted a great
deal of press attention and the organisers even received a telegram of
support from the Queen. The aims of the Association (later named the
National Childbirth Association and now the National Childbirth Trust –
NCT) were to teach pregnant women skills in relaxation, breathing and
massage and to build up their confidence through emotional support. It
rapidly became clear that the second aim could be achieved only through
the setting up of groups in which women could discuss their anxieties
and share information. Jessica Dick Read, Sheila Kitzinger and Betty
Parsons were among the first to set up what would become known as
antenatal classes. A small fee was charged for these classes, which were
usually held in the teacher's own home.[59] All teachers supplemented their
own experience of childbirth by completing the training course
developed by the Trust.

The NCT continued Read's emphasis on the pregnant woman and
her needs – particularly her emotional needs–and it was this that led to
the perception that those associated with the Trust were hostile to the
medical profession. In fact, during the 1960s the NCT proceeded
cautiously in its efforts to modify obstetric practice. It invited leading
obstetricians to serve on its advisory panel and sought, in Margery
Tew's words, 'co-operation and complementing rather than confronta-
tion between providers and users'.[60] It was not until the 1970s that it
was forced to adopt a less conciliatory approach, largely as a result of
ever-increasing levels of intervention in childbirth and a soaring rate of
induced labour. None the less, books like Sheila Kitzinger's *The
Experience of Childbirth* (1964) certainly challenged and were intended
to challenge both conventional obstetric practice and wider social
attitudes to the pregnant woman.

In this best-seller, Kitzinger drew on her experience as an anthropologist and on contemporary psychology to explore the social and psychological aspects of pregnancy and childbirth, concentrating on the woman rather than what Read had called the 'reproductory machine'. Like Read, she links physical process and spiritual feeling, arguing that childbirth is not simply the means of getting a baby out of one's body but involves one's relationship to life as a whole, 'the part one plays in the order of things'. Pregnancy, too, she argues, has for some women a markedly spiritual dimension: 'as the baby develops and can be felt moving inside, to some women annunciation, incarnation, seem to become facts of their own existence'.[61] Rather like Byatt, Kitzinger contrasts this uplifting potential with the grim realities which face women as soon as they are sucked into the machinery of antenatal care. When they visit the antenatal clinic they face a wait of up to three hours in gloomy and sometimes dirty rooms, with large numbers of other pregnant women. They are examined on a high, hard table by a doctor who 'prods and pushes and presses his hand painfully into the woman's groin and finally slides his fingers into her vagina. He rarely tells her that everything is all right, but looks grave and preoccupied and leaves her to imagine the worst' (p. 49).

In such circumstances, Kitzinger argues, some woman may resist pregnancy and such resistance can take the form of depression. Kitzinger here uses the language of psychology to describe what could be read as a twentieth-century version of the 'insanity of pregnancy'. She points out that the field of the psychological care of pregnant woman is still 'a vast and unexplored' one. In her experience, some women feel depression because they feel 'humiliated or trapped by their pregnancy'. Moreover, at a stage in pregnancy between 34 and 37 weeks many women suffer 'unaccountable depression', with their self-confidence being at a very low ebb. Depression prior to the birth is a mental state which should be foreseen and attended to: Kitzinger writes that it is 'much more common than the depression which follows childbirth on or about the third day after, which one hears so much about' (p. 57). Although depression in pregnancy is mentioned in contemporary obstetric textbooks, it is most often linked with obvious triggers such as illegitimacy: Kitzinger is one of the few writers to engage in detail with the psychological effects of pregnancy.[62] Thus she writes about the revulsion which some women feel when they think of the child within: 'They feel physically nauseated by the body of the child developing within them like a parasite, drawing life from them. They feel horrified by the inevitability of the process once it has

started, horrified at the thickening of their bodies and at the movements of the kicking baby' (p. 53). She describes too fears of abnormality and monstrosity: 'What if this thing I am nourishing and
cherishing within my own body, around which my whole life is built
now, whose pulse beats fast deep within me – what if this child should
prove to be a hideous deformed creature, sub-human, a thing I should
be able to love, but which I would shudder to see?' (p. 57). In linking
such fears with the mother's own psychology, and with feelings of
inadequacy or guilt which are common, Kitzinger goes some way
towards defusing them.

This was, perhaps, the more necessary in the light of the exploration in contemporary popular fiction of the possibility of xenogenesis, a term coined by Julian Huxley to denote the gestation of a
creature genetically unrelated to its mother. This idea is most memo-
rably presented in John Wyndham's novel *The Midwich Cuckoos*
(1957). Wyndham creates a scenario in which the sleepy English
village of Midwich is visited by aliens from another planet, and in
one night the entire child-bearing population becomes pregnant with
alien children. When the children are born it gradually becomes clear
that they are not only alien but telepathic. The question thus arises
as to whether the thirty or so girls and thirty or so boys can be considered as individuals or whether they should be considered as the
several parts of, respectively, one female super-spirit and one male
super-spirit. The appearance of the children can be interpreted in the
light of contemporary anxieties about the Atomic Bomb, delinquent
children and 'unmarried mothers', a category which was causing
concern because the burden of supporting such mothers and their
children now fell on the Welfare State rather than on individual families and/or charities. The novel can also be read in psychoanalytic
terms as representing male fear of what Barbara Creed has called the
fantasy of 'the parthenogenic, archaic mother ... the being who exists
prior to knowledge of the phallus'.[63] Through the character of the
novelist Gordon Zellaby, Wyndham presents a view of women as sub-
limely indifferent to male concerns: 'Men may build and destroy and
play with all their toys; they are uncomfortable nuisances, ephemeral
conveniences, mere scamperers-about, while woman, in mystical
umbilical connexion with the great tree of life itself, *knows* that she is
indispensable.'[64] The use of the umbilical metaphor to link women
with the origins of life suggests both fear and longing for Creed's
'generative, parthenogenic mother – that ancient archaic figure who
gives birth to all living things'.

However, the novel explores not just male fear of women's monstrous power (expressed in the alien births) but also female anxieties in relation to 'incubating' the alien. Echoing some of the feelings described by Kitzinger, one of the women indicates that the invasion of her body has taken away her sense of human identity: '"Not to *know*," she exclaimed. "To know there's something growing there – and not to be sure how, or what. It's so – so abasing, Gordon. It makes me feel like an animal"' (p. 73). These pregnancies thus encode a number of interrelated fears, which include fear of individual reproductive failure as well as fear of the annihilation of the human race.

Wyndham also anticipates some of the social and ethical issues which were to arise in relation to surrogate pregnancy. For example, some of the women of the village remain attached to 'their' children even though there is no biological or genetic link between them. Zellaby explains, 'They all *know* well enough now that, biologically speaking, they are not even their own children, but they did have the trouble and pain of bearing them – and that … isn't the kind of link they can just snip and forget' (p. 156). Ethical and legal issues which were to arise in connection with human cloning are also anticipated, as Zellaby and others struggle with the question of whether the identical children should be treated, in law, as analogous to individual human beings. Wyndham's novel is thus prescient. It was becoming clear to many in the post-war period that some forms of reproductive technology would become viable sooner rather than later, and would change irrevocably the nature and scope of reproductive medicine.

5
Reproductive Futures

Second-wave feminism and reproduction

While first-wave feminism had brought about women's political enfranchisement and had strengthened their legal rights, second-wave feminism developed out of the recognition that gender inequality was perpetuated as much by the power of ideology as by political and legal structures. The second wave thus went beyond campaigning for material change and began to explore and challenge dominant ideological representations of femininity. Apart from the construction of woman as sex-object (critiqued most famously in the 1968 Miss America 'bra burning' protest), the most entrenched ideological construction was that of woman-as-homemaker, the twentieth-century version of Coventry Patmore's 'Angel in the House'. Both the ideological construction and material determinants of such femininity came under attack, and from a bewildering variety of positions, for second-wave feminism was anything but uniform.

One of the issues on which there was the greatest divergence of opinion was that of women's relationship to reproduction. In *The Dialectic of Sex*, first published in 1970, the radical feminist Shulamith Firestone took the uncompromising line that women's reproductive power was a primary reason for their subordination and that they would only be free when this reproductive burden was lifted from them. Agreeing with Simone de Beauvoir that biological differences did not in themselves necessitate the domination of women by men, she none the less contended that 'the reproductive *functions* of these differences' made such domination inevitable.[1] Accordingly, she demanded 'the freeing of women from the tyranny of their reproductive biology by every means available, and the diffusion of the childbearing and childrearing role to the society as a whole, men as well as women' (p. 233). Such a demand was predicated on the assumption that technology would shortly provide reliable contraception, artificial insemination and an artificial placenta to which the embryo could be transferred early in gestation. Thus, 'the reproduction of the species by one sex for the benefit of both would be replaced by (at least the option of) artificial reproduction' (p. 12).

Firestone thus recruits the scientific control of reproduction (earlier viewed with ambivalence by the Haldanes) firmly for the feminist political cause. For Firestone, women's liberation can be brought about only through the control of nature, but scientific advances do not in themselves guarantee this: what matters is the use to which such advances are put. As she puts it, 'though man is increasingly capable of freeing himself from the biological conditions that created his tyranny over women and children, he has little reason to want to give this tyranny up' (pp.10–11). Thus she argues that, by analogy with the proletariat in the Marxist model of revolution, women must free themselves by seizing control of the means of reproduction, including the new technologies and the social institutions of childbearing and childrearing. Here Firestone anticipates the male domination of the new reproductive technologies which has recently been critiqued by Germaine Greer and others.[2]

Socialist feminists, by contrast, resisted such an understanding of reproduction as natural and pre-cultural. They argued that it was the cultural separation of production and reproduction which was the primary cause of women's oppression. As Susan Himmelweit put it in *Feminist Review*:

Production (or much of it anyway) is a social activity, under the control of capital, socially valued and distributed through the price of its products and for which workers are paid a wage. Reproduction (in the sense of having babies) is a private activity with no direct control by capital, no social mechanism for its recognition and co-ordination, and for which no recompense is paid to women.[3]

For socialist feminists like Himmelweit, it was crucial that the separation of reproduction from production was seen as a cultural construction and, as such, amenable to change. Juliet Mitchell similarly attempted to reconcile socialist and feminist perspectives and argued for the need to challenge existing family structures which naturalised patriarchal exploitation of the reproductive woman.[4] The liberal feminist Janet Radcliffe Richards challenged, in turn, socialist feminist attempts to reintegrate production and reproduction, the public and private spheres. Radcliffe Richards took particular exception to the socialist feminist view that motherhood constituted a social contribution which should be recognised and financially recompensed. With a fine disregard for the complex and varying circumstances in which children are conceived, she argued that 'children do not just appear out of nowhere; they are born because the parents want them' and that 'there seems no reason at all for children to be subsidised by the state, because children are not a kind of external drain on the parents' income, but a chosen way of spending it'.[5]

Radical and socialist feminists thus wished to 'diffuse', as Firestone put it, the burden of reproduction through a wider society, whereas liberals such as Radcliffe Richards more cautiously supported assistance for individual women who had been exploited in relation to reproduction. The most influential Anglo-American feminist analysis of reproduction takes a different line again. In *Of Woman Born* (published in 1976 in the US and a year later in Britain), Adrienne Rich famously distinguishes between motherhood as an experience and motherhood as an institution. Like radical and socialist feminists, she offers a critique of motherhood as it has been constructed in patriarchal society: this has 'withheld over one-half the human species from the decisions affecting their lives; it exonerates men from fatherhood in any authentic sense'.[6] However, Rich builds on her sense of the 'potential relationship' of women to their powers of reproduction to suggest a way forward which does not involve women's lives becoming, as she would see it, closer to those of men through the deployment of reproductive technologies and shared childcare arrangements. Rather, Rich suggests that women should uncover a feminine identity rooted in the corporeal, which has been occluded by patriarchal control of discursive and social formations. She writes:

> In arguing that we have by no means yet explored or understood our biological grounding, the miracle and paradox of the female body and its spiritual and political meanings, I am really asking whether women cannot begin, at last, to *think through the body*, to connect what has been so cruelly disorganized ... There is for the first time today a possibility of converting our physicality into both knowledge and power. (p. 284)

Rich sees women's physiology as grounding a specifically feminine subjectivity and creativity. Her arguments are utopian and also dangerous, for they tread a fine line between envisaging the new and returning women to fixed interpretations of biological difference.

While Anglo-American feminists concentrated on the social contexts of reproduction, French feminists approached the subject from a psychoanalytic point of view. The most powerful analysis from this perspective is that of Julia Kristeva, who published three influential essays in the 1970s. 'Motherhood According to Giovanni Bellini' was first published in 1975 and translated into English in 1979; 'Stabat Mater' was first published in 1977 and translated into English in 1987; and 'Women's Time' was first published in 1979 and translated into English in 1981. In all three essays Kristeva focuses on the subjective experience of pregnancy, arguing that it is a state/process which exists on the border between nature and culture. In 'Motherhood According to Giovanni Bellini' she examines the discourses which are currently available for the understanding of pregnancy. She argues that the discourse of science cannot accommodate the split subjectivity of the pregnant woman; it can only construe the pregnant woman as either subject to or master of a natural, pre-social, biological process. If she is subject to this process, over which she has no control, her identity as a speaking subject is threatened. If, alternatively, she is positioned as controlling the process, she is still heavily implicated in the pre-social and pre-symbolic, and again her identity as a speaking subject is undermined. By contrast, Kristeva argues that Christianity does address the move from nature to culture in the maternal body through the image of the Virgin Mary. However, the image of the Virgin also fails fully to comprehend the bodily meaning of maternity, for 'theology defines maternity only as an impossible elsewhere, a sacred beyond'.[7]

Kristeva's account of the divided subjectivity of the pregnant woman rests on her understanding of embryonic and foetal development as necessarily eluding representation yet apprehended by the mother, who is thus split between the natural/pre-symbolic and the cultural/symbolic. It is this splitting which creates a vertiginous sense of pleasure and pain, as the opening passage of 'Stabat Mater', invoking Kristeva's own experience of pregnancy, suggests:

FLASH – instant of time or of dream without time; inordinately swollen atoms of a bond, a vision, a shiver, a yet formless, unnameable embryo. Epiphanies. Photos of what is not yet visible and that language necessarily skims over from afar, allusively. Words that are always too distant, too abstract for this underground swarming of seconds, folding in unimaginable spaces.[8]

Kristeva's analysis of pregnancy challenges Freud's masculinist view of the baby as a penis-substitute. Rather, she links the desire for a child with the desire to return to the maternal body. Pregnancy and birth offer the possibility of reunion with the mother and a return to primal homosexual bonds: 'By giving birth, the woman enters into contact with her mother; she becomes, she is her own mother; they are the same continuity differentiating itself' (p. 303).

For Kristeva, in its approach to the pre-symbolic and pre-social, pregnancy is a risky experience. In 'Women's Time' she describes it as 'a dramatic ordeal: a splitting of the body, the division and coexistence of self and other, of nature and awareness, of physiology and speech ... Pregnancy is a sort of institutionalized, socialized, and natural psychosis'.[9] None the less, she argues that pregnancy can offer a model for a new understanding of identity and of inter-subjective relations. Neither the mother nor the foetus controls pregnancy and neither is a unified subject. The experience of pregnancy can thus offer a template for what Kristeva calls a 'herethics', based on a more fluid understanding of inter-subjective bonds. The reformulation of contemporary ethics, she thus contends,

> demands the contribution of women: Of women who harbor the desire to reproduce (to have stability). Of women who are available so that our speaking species, which knows it is mortal, might withstand death. Of mothers. For an heretical ethics separated from morality, an *herethics*, is perhaps no more than that which in life makes bonds, thoughts, and therefore the thought of death, bearable. (p. 330)

The feminist philosopher Iris Young builds on Kristeva's work in her influential essay 'Pregnant Embodiment: Subjectivity and Alienation'. Working outside the psychoanalytic framework employed by Kristeva, Young none the less suggests, similarly, that the pregnant subject is 'decentred, split, or doubled in several ways'.[10] Thus she argues that a description of pregnant embodiment can constitute a significant philosophical intervention, extending and challenging contemporary thinking about subjectivity and bodily identity. Young focuses particularly on the existential phenomenology of thinkers such as Maurice Merleau-Ponty, arguing that while phenomenology to some extent breaks with Cartesian dualism by locating consciousness and subjectivity within the body, it still assumes the unity of the subject and thus a separation between subject and object. Pregnant embodiment undoes this dichotomy: 'Pregnancy challenges the integration of my body experience by rendering fluid the boundary between what is within, myself, and what is outside, separate. I experience my insides as the space of another, yet my own body' (p. 409). Moreover, phenomenology maintains a distinction between transcendence and immanence as two modes of bodily being. Thus it is assumed that, in so far as one acts effectively in the world, one is not aware of one's body: only in sickness or fatigue does one become aware of the body as immanent matter. Again, pregnant embodiment dissolves this distinction, for as Young writes:

> Pregnancy roots me to the earth, makes me conscious of the physicality of my body *not as an object*, but as the material weight that I am in movement ... In pregnancy this fact of existence never leaves me. I am an actor transcending through each moment to further projects, but the solid inertia and demands of my body call me to my limits not as an obstacle to action, but only as a fleshy relation to the earth. (pp. 411–12; emphasis added)

As Young is careful to point out, such sophisticated reflection on pregnant embodiment depends on pregnancy's being a choice, undertaken with adequate emotional and financial resources. As she notes, 'most women in human history have not chosen their pregnancies in this sense ... So I speak in large measure for an experience that must be instituted and for those pregnant women who have been able to take up their situation as their own' (p. 408). However, the second section of her essay addresses issues that affect many women, regardless of the extra-medical context of their pregnancies. Young contends that the pregnant subject's encounter with contemporary obstetric medicine increasingly alienates her from her own experience. The deployment of technology such as foetal heart monitors and real-time ultrasound transfers control over the means of observing pregnancy from the woman to the medical professionals. Thus, the pregnant woman's 'unique knowledge of her body processes and the life of the fetus ... is reduced in value, replaced by more objective means of observation' (p. 416). Young's argument recalls Martha Mears' eighteenth-century invocation of the 'mysterious consent' between mother and foetus, discussed in chapter 1, which endows the mother with a peculiarly direct knowledge of foetal movement and development. Young goes on to argue that a basic condition of good medical practice is that the physician and patient share the same lived-body experience. Yet pregnancy and childbirth entail 'a unique body subjectivity that is difficult to empathize with unless one is or has been pregnant', and since the vast majority of obstetricians are men, this basic condition of good therapeutic practice cannot be met in obstetrics (p. 416). Again, this recalls the arguments of eighteenth-century writers such as Elizabeth Nihell, who suggested that female medical attendants had 'a kind of intuitive guide within themselves', which enabled them to understand the situation of the pregnant woman better than rival male practitioners.[11]

Fay Weldon's novel *Puffball* (1980) engages with a number of these issues, explicitly locating pregnancy on the border between nature and culture. The novel focuses primarily on the subjectivity of the pregnant Liffey (her name recalling the river Liffey which winds through Dublin and which is identified in Joyce's *Finnegan's Wake* with Anna Livia Plurabelle, mother and source of life). Liffey's understanding of her pregnancy is juxtaposed with that of a number of other characters and of a dramatised narrator. Liffey frames her pregnancy primarily in terms of nature, which she conceives as a beneficent force creating rhythms and cycles of being which are 'natural' in the sense of being fitting and appropriate. It is this desire to be at one with 'the rhythms of nature' which, she thinks, has drawn her to live in the country and agree to have a child. When she becomes pregnant, however, she discovers that she knows 'next to nothing about pregnancy, or what went on inside her, and really had no particular wish to know', and she refuses all knowledge of what the narrator calls the 'bloody, pulpy, incoherent, surging mass of pulsing organs within'.[12]

Her conception of the natural (unlike that of Kristeva) excludes the bloody and the incoherent, and remains an idealisation and indeed an abstraction. She feels that she wants 'to be a woman like other women; to feel herself part of nature's process: to subdue the individual spirit to some greater whole. When, now, she knelt in the flower beds and crumbled the earth ... she felt she was the servant of Nature's kingdom, and not its mistress' (p. 156). Liffey thus locates herself as immersed in/subject to nature, but it is an idealised nature. She oscillates between her sense of being immersed in bodily process and an effort to construct and retain the subjective meaning of her experience, which she construes in terms of natural religion. Her experience of annunciation is thus expressed in these terms:

Liffey sat on the ground and turned her face towards the mild sun. She felt a presence: the touch of a spirit, clear and benign. She opened her eyes, startled, but there was no one there, only a dazzle in the sky where the sun struck slantwise between the few puffy white clouds which hovered over the Tor.

'It's me,' said the spirit, said the baby, 'I'm here. I have arrived. You are perfectly all right, and so am I. Don't worry.' The words were spoken in her head: they were graceful, and certain. They charmed. (p. 139)

While Liffey interprets her pregnancy in terms deriving from natural religion, or white magic, her neighbour, Mabs, attempts to stall the pregnancy through witchcraft. Mabs is jealous of Liffey, partly because she thinks, with some reason, that the baby could be her husband's. She believes that she can do Liffey harm by 'overlooking' her and by the administration of potions such as ergot in elderberry wine. While ill-wishing may have no effect, ergot is a well-known abortifacient and, as the narrator points out, women such as Mabs draw on a store of effective knowledge which overlaps with that of the medical profession: 'The drugs [Mabs] prepared – as her mother's before her – were the same as the local doctor had to offer; psychoactive agents, prophylactics, antiseptics, narcotics, hypnotics, anaesthetics and antibiotics' (p. 25). Mabs, however, uses these drugs in overdose, not to restore 'natural body chemistry'. By contrast, the local doctor does not wish Liffey ill, but the text foregrounds the way in which his perspective on Liffey, different in so many ways from that of Mabs, none the less diminishes the pregnant woman in ways that hers does not. Seeing Liffey through the lens of clinical practice, Dr Southey identifies her with the animal and pre-social: 'He wished he could keep his respect for pregnant women. They seemed to him to belong so completely to the animal kingdom that it was almost strange to hear them talk' (p. 169). His clinical views are supplemented by a scientific commentary on the pregnancy supplied at intervals by the narrator. Thus at sixteen weeks the reader is told: 'The baby weighed five ounces and was six inches long. It had limbs with working joints, and finger and toes, each with its completing nail. It was clearly male. It lay curled in its amniotic sac, legs crossed, knees up towards its lowered head, which it sheltered with little arms' (p. 166). Despite the anthropomorphic attitude to the foetus in this 'scientific' account, it elides completely the subjectivity of the pregnant woman.

None the less it is scientific medicine in the form of an emergency Caesarean which saves both Liffey and her baby, despite her failure to make arrangements to get to hospital quickly after placenta praevia has been diagnosed. Thus, while the novel acknowledges the inadequacies of 'human relations in obstetrics' and gives full weight to the pregnant woman's need to construct her own narrative, it is plotted in such a way as to foreground the fact that instrumental and institutionalised medicine saves lives. It is the doctor's knowledge which leads him to suspect placenta praevia and a hospital ultrasound scan which confirms this – a scan taken against Liffey's wishes, as she feels that the ultrasound picture represents 'an untimely manifestation of spirit into flesh' (p. 194). And finally it is the doctor, on call to another patient, who finds Liffey walking along a lane in a trail of blood and drives her to hospital for her Caesarean section. The text can thus be read as a tart rejoinder to those who reject any kind of medical intervention in pregnancy on the grounds that it is 'unnatural'. The sub-plot of the novel confirms this: one of the women staying in Liffey's old flat is encouraged by her elder sister to have nothing to do with the medical profession ('an essential part of the male conspiracy against women') during pregnancy. When her labour begins she is first ignored, then inappropriately drugged by her sister and eventually gives birth to a stillborn child.

Foetal persons, foetal patients

A number of feminist critics have argued that the construction of the foetus-as-person has been inextricably bound up with the development and use of foetal imagery.[13] The age of the foetal portrait was inaugurated with the publication in *Life* magazine in 1965 of Lars Nilsson's dramatic photographs of the embryo in the womb. The cover photograph was rapidly circulated round the world, and Nilsson's book, *A Child Is Born: The Drama of Life before Birth*, which used many of the images in the *Life* magazine issue, attracted widespread publicity. The first English-language edition of the book was published in 1966, with revised editions in 1977 and 1990. Ostensibly, it interleaves and establishes connections between two pictorial narratives, one an 'objective' scientific record of embryonic/foetal development, the other a social narrative of pregnancy in the context of middle-class family life. However, as Sandra Matthews and Laura Wexler have pointed out, neither narrative is objective, and each has been constructed with great care to convey specific cultural meanings.[14] Thus, while the image used on the cover of *Life* was indeed, as was claimed, 'the first portrait ever made of a living embryo inside its mother's womb', *all* the other images were of embryos which had been 'surgically removed from the womb': in other words, they were dead.[15] Thus, rather as with William

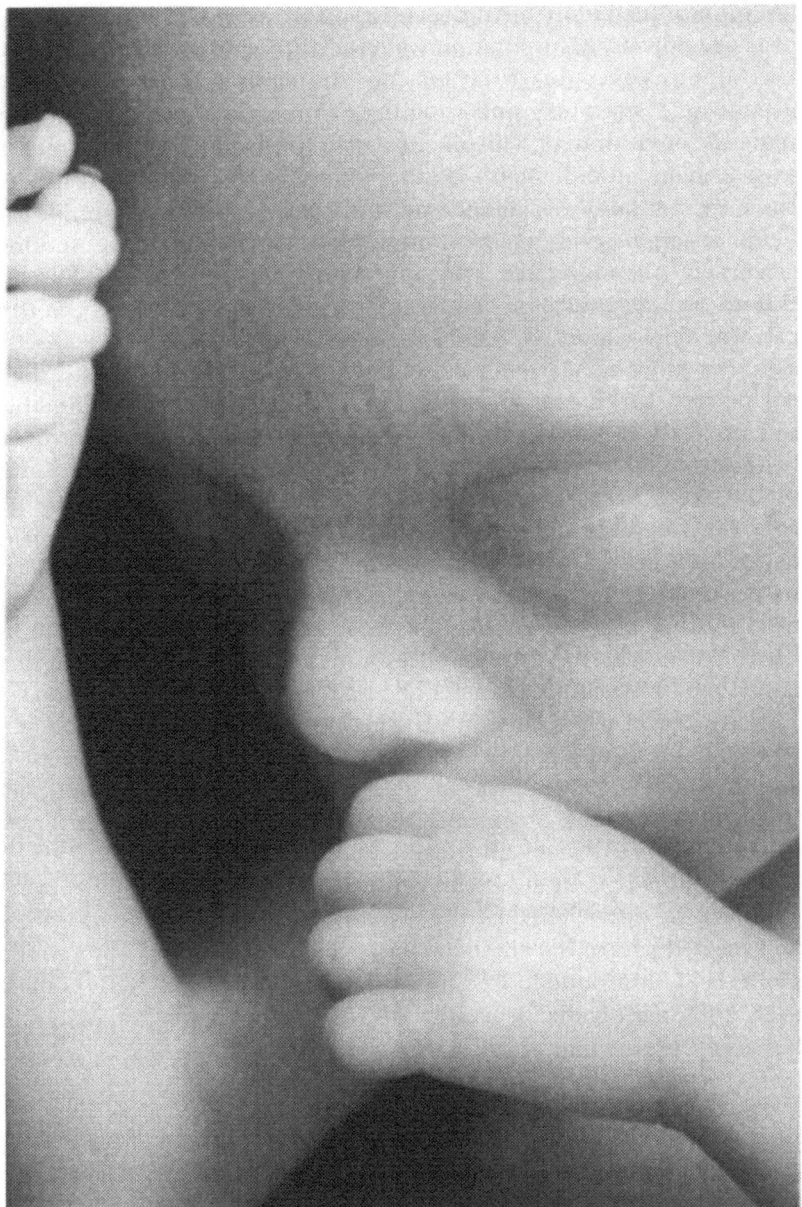

Figure 5   Lars Nilsson, 20-week foetus sucking thumb. Wellcome Photo Library.

Hunter in the eighteenth century, this new technique for the representation of life before birth depended on the technical manipulation of dead subjects. Manipulation was crucial too in the construction of the famous cover image. By placing the embryo against the background of a starry sky and isolating it almost completely from the maternal environment, Nilsson created an iconic image of the embryo as spaceman, a heroic figure of pure potential. The physical reality of the maternal body was elided and in its place was a figuration of the womb as empty space, ready for inscription and colonisation. Another celebrated Nilsson image, the photograph of a foetus sucking its thumb, also depended on the careful use of photo-technology, in this case the deployment of light and shade, to construct a 'fake' foetal skin. For as Imogen Tyler has pointed out, although the foetus does not develop a skin until a late stage in development, 'it must nonetheless be imaged photographically as having a skin in order to be imagined as a discrete being': skin is a part of personhood. Tyler sums up the effect of such visual moves: 'the visibility of the foetus, who has been bestowed the status of a subject by fact of this visual "independence", is achieved at the cost of the increasing invisibility of the pregnant woman as the actual subject of gestation'.[16] It is only relatively recently that this 'invisibility' has been contested by artists such as Chris Nurse, who has created ultrasound portraits foregrounding the enmeshed indivisibility of maternal and foetal bodies.

In the period when Nilsson's foetal portraits were being circulated, real-time ultrasound scanners were also becoming available in the UK and, by the late 1970s, ultrasound scans were being offered routinely to pregnant women at around 16 weeks' gestation. It is currently offered at 11–13 weeks and again at 18–20 weeks, and though in clinical terms it is by no means clear that the costs of such routine scanning are outweighed by the benefits, it has none the less become an expected part of the antenatal package.[17] As noted in chapter 4, the pioneers of ultrasound looked forward to its social as well as its clinical uses, anticipating that it would offer the opportunity for maternal bonding with the unborn child. However, as Iris Young has argued, the scan is often experienced in terms of alienation.

One difficulty is that ultrasound technology by its nature invokes the idea of the 'foetal spaceman'. Ultrasound pictures show a figure unconstrained by gravity, depicted via the same medium as was used to transmit the first pictures of man on the moon. By association of ideas, such an image may well seem like that of an alien being. A sense of detachment and alienation may also be reinforced through the physical

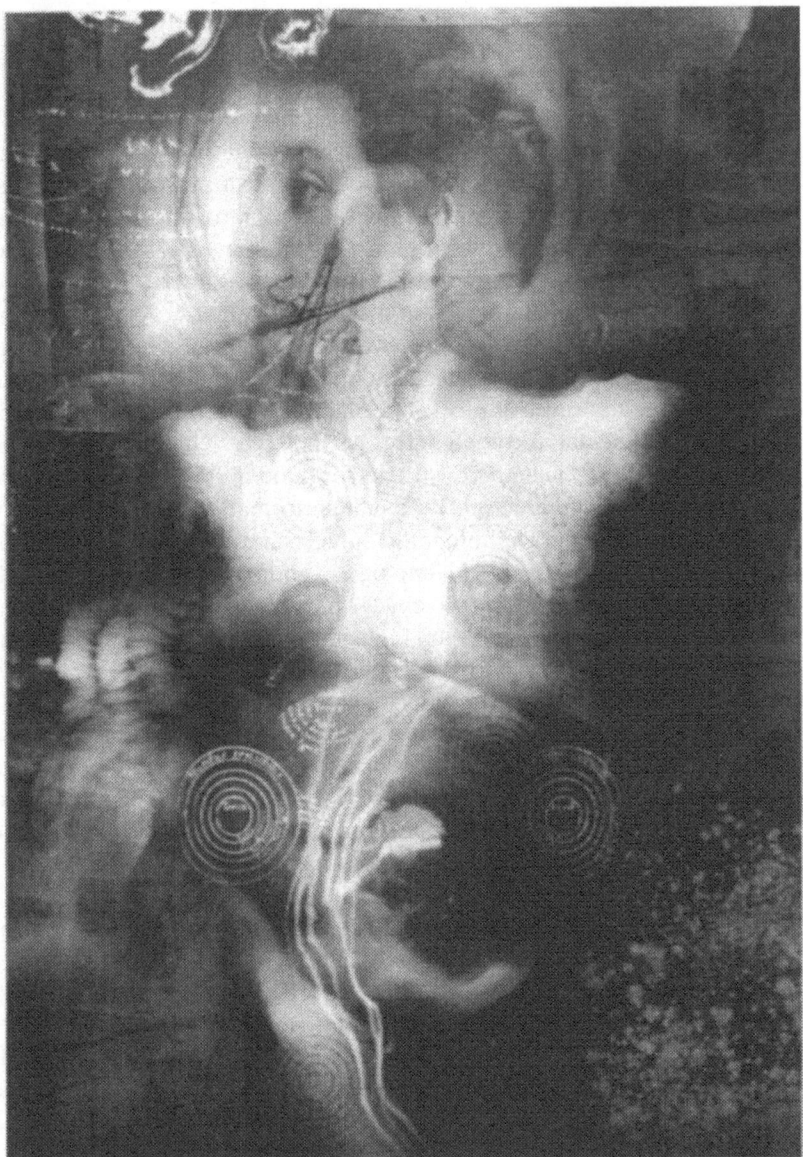

Figure 6   Pregnancy artwork. Chris Nurse/Wellcome Photo Library.

setting of the scan, as the visual image appears on a monitor detached from the mother's body, often several metres away. Thus, as with the Nilsson portraits, images which construct an apparently 'independent' foetal person – and which invite social investment in that person – may have the effect of alienating the one being who has an intimate, but apparently disregarded, bodily connection with the child.

As Rosalind Petchesky has argued in her influential essay on ultra-sound, it is impossible to generalise about the meaning of foetal images. Noting that 'from their beginning, such photographs have represented the foetus as primary and autonomous, the woman as absent or periph-eral', and exploring the way in which foetal images have been deployed in a number of campaigns by the pro-life movement, Petchesky con-tends none the less that pregnant women do not easily give up their own rights of interpretation over such images.[18] Thus their response to a scan will depend on the clinical context and setting, but also more cru-cially on their social and ideological perspectives. They may resist the tendency to invest the embryo with personhood if, for example, they are at risk of miscarriage or suspect a foetal abnormality. It should thus by no means be assumed that pregnant subjects are the passive victims of reproductive technologies or ideologies. Following Petchesky's lead, many feminist commentators in the US have investigated and critiqued the ideological uses made of foetal imagery, but less attention has been paid to this subject in Britain, where the anti-abortion lobby is less pow-erful. However, it could be argued that in the UK foetal imagery has seeped into popular consciousness in a more insidious manner. The ultrasound scan has become widely accepted as a crucial rite of passage in pregnancy, the point at which the embryo becomes (at 11–13 weeks) a 'real baby'. In Jane Green's popular novel *Babyville*, for example, the ultrasound functions in precisely this manner:

> We're both staring at the screen, and I don't know what the sono-grapher's talking about because I can't see anything at all other than a greenish tunnel, and suddenly my heart flips over and Mark and I gasp, squeezing each other's hands tightly.
>
> 'Oh, my God!' we whisper in unison. 'Did you see that?' And sud-denly the screen becomes clear. There is a tiny leg kicking up in the air, and we follow the leg up as we start to define the shape of a baby. My baby. Our baby. A living being inside of me.[19]

Such a view of the 13-week embryo as a 'baby' (reinforced rhetorically by repetition) carries a strong ideological charge which is not helpful to those who support unpressured abortion choice.

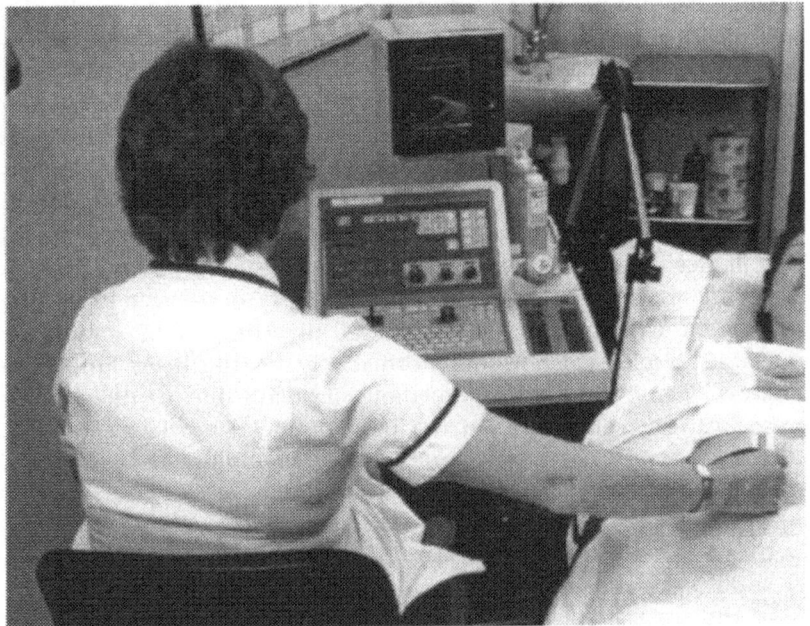

Figure 7 Ultrasound scanning equipment. Wellcome Photo Library.

If foetal imagery has worked to construct the idea of the foetus as a 'person' representative in some senses of the future of a society, this tendency has been reinforced by an ever-increasing increasing interest in and understanding of foetal physiology. In 1972 a study was published in *The Lancet* which confirmed for the first time the existence of independent foetal breathing, and much subsequent research has focused on the distinctive neurological, circulatory and respiratory systems of the foetus.[20] In making certain – albeit limited – therapeutic interventions possible, such research has led to the construction of the foetus as both person and patient. This perspective has far-reaching implications for our understanding of the pregnant body: if it is accepted, the pregnant body must be considered as a site which contains, or grounds, two persons, whose interests may not always coincide. In such circumstances the question must arise: whose interests have priority, those of the mother or those of the foetus? As Alexander McCall Smith has argued, there are two sets of circumstances in which the interests of the mother and the foetus may be said to conflict.[21] The first are those in which the 'general behaviour' of the mother has the effect of harming the foetus. Such behaviour might include heavy smoking and drinking or drug abuse, and might also include 'lifestyle' choices such as sleeping rough and not eating properly. In the earlier twentieth century, when the dominant model of pregnancy was that of the foetus as successful parasite, such behaviour would not have been thought particularly dangerous. However, as noted in the introduction, recent research has posited a more competitive model of the relation between mother and foetus. In relation to nutrition, for example, it is now known that the foetus cannot take all that it needs from the mother in times of scarcity. If the foetus is receiving an inadequate supply of nutrients or oxygen from the mother, it will have to make choices, diverting to the brain, for example, blood which would normally go to the liver, lungs and kidneys. While this has an immediate survival value, it will compromise future development. In the light of such knowledge, there is increasing pressure on pregnant women to modify their lifestyle. Rachel Cusk describes this regulatory pressure in *A Life's Work*:

> Like a bad parent, the literature of pregnancy bristles with threats and the promise of reprisal, with ghoulish hints at the consequences of thoughtless actions ...*When you raise your fork to your lips*, reads one book on this subject, *look at it and think, Is this the best bite I can give my baby? If the answer is no, put your fork down.*[22]

As Cusk indicates, it is the literature of pregnancy (which now includes not only 'advice' books but magazines such as *Pregnancy* and *You and Your Baby*) which exerts this ideological pressure. However, in legal terms in Britain the pregnant woman remains free to act in a way that compromises the foetus if she wishes to do so. In cases which have been brought to test this issue, the view has been taken that maternal liberty, and the right to maintain one's bodily integrity, should take precedence over the rights of the foetus. In the case of *Re F (in utero)* (1988), for example, an attempt was made to make a foetus a ward of court in order for social workers to control maternal behaviour which, in their view, threatened the foetus. The court rejected this, ruling in favour of the maternal interest in freedom.[23] As McCall Smith points out, the ethical issues in such cases are complex. While it can be argued that the mother has an 'absolute obligation' not to engage in harmful conduct directed exclusively to the harming of the foetus, the issue is less clear-cut when she engages in such conduct because it gives her pleasure. It might be argued that her freedom should in this case be subordinated to 'the interest of the fetus in a healthy future'; alternatively it could be argued that the mother's interest should take priority because it alone is capable of being ascertained. Some would deny that foetal interest exists at all, because the foetus lacks awareness of its interest (p. 165).

The other circumstances in which the interests of mother and foetus may be said to conflict are those in which the mother refuses medical treatment which would be beneficial to the foetus. Such cases have been brought to court in the US, where a ruling was made that a compulsory blood transfusion should be administered to a woman in the eighth month of pregnancy; she had refused a transfusion on religious grounds. In other cases, maternal opposition to Caesarean section has been overridden in the interests of the foetus. No such rulings have been made in Britain, and the decisions taken in the US must be seen in the light of a different political culture, in which there is a great deal of public concern over abortion rights. In such circumstances, the right of the unborn child to therapeutic intervention may be defended as part of a wider pro-life agenda. However, although the climate of opinion is different in Britain, there is concern here over the impact of developments in the US. As Cusk notes: 'I read newspaper reports of women in America being prosecuted for harming their unborn foetuses and wonder how this can be; how the body can become a public space, like a telephone box, that can unlawfully vandalise itself. It is my fear of authority, of conformity, that is pricked by such stories' (p. 34).

The concept of the 'foetal patient' brings with it another possibility, that a child might be considered to have a legal claim against its mother in relation to her conduct during pregnancy. No such claim has yet been brought in Britain, but the emergence of the foetus as a separate person, with accompanying rights, raises the possibility of legal protection for rights which could be claimed retrospectively. As McCall Smith points out, such a vision 'is alien to the human, one flesh, notion of motherhood which has traditionally informed moral thinking in this area' (p. 170). However, medical and technical developments, including a wide range of new reproductive technologies, are putting increasing pressure on this 'one flesh' model of pregnancy.

New reproductive technologies

Although we have not yet achieved the degree of control over reproduction anticipated by many twentieth-century thinkers, there have been rapid advances over the last three decades. One field in which there have been significant developments is that of antenatal screening. In addition to ultrasound scanning, serum screening tests are now available at 16–18 weeks which measure the levels of alpha-fetoprotein (AFP) in the blood and can be used to assess the risk of having a baby with spina bifida. Amniocentesis can also detect such abnormalities, but is not offered routinely as it involves a small risk of miscarriage. Similarly, chorionic villus sampling (CVS) can detect inherited disorders such as Down's syndrome and sickle-cell anaemia but is offered only to women at high risk, as it too carries some risk of miscarriage. The advent of such techniques has inevitably created ethical dilemmas for both patients and medical practitioners. In response, a technique of 'non-directive' counselling has been developed to support patients post-diagnosis. Non-directiveness is seen as crucial in genetic counselling because of the perceived need to distinguish the contemporary field of genetics (developing out of the discovery of DNA) from the historical field of eugenics. Eugenics is associated with coercion by a dominant social group, whereas genetics seeks to present itself in terms of individual choice. None the less, research has shown that many of those involved in genetic counselling find it difficult to maintain a non-directive stance, not least because patients may have a strong desire for guidance as well as for information. As the authors of one research paper put it, 'patients ... may not always want to control what happens to them, the priority being to maintain choice, which may include the choice to relinquish control to another person'.[24]

Moreover, it has been argued that 'non-directiveness' in genetic counselling is not only impossible to achieve, but that clinging to an ethos of 'value-neutrality' in such circumstances may mean that public debate about the issues is stifled.[25] The need for debate about the new genetics has become more urgent with the development of screening techniques associated with IVF technology. In cases where prospective parents carry heritable diseases, it is now possible for embryos to be created by IVF and screened so that only those unaffected by the disease are implanted. For example, if the heritable disease is haemophilia, which affects only males, female embryos only can be implanted. A more complex case has arisen recently in which the parents of a child in urgent need of a bone marrow transplant wished to have another child by IVF to act as a donor (there was no other source of compatible bone marrow). The case caused controversy because it was argued that, if the procedure were allowed, a child would be created as a means to an end, not for its own sake. The UK Human Fertilisation and Embryology Authority ruled against the parents, but their decision was overturned on appeal to the European Court. Dame Mary Warnock, the original architect of the HFEA, has recently written that she can see no objection to such a procedure, as the baby who would be born would be loved for itself, not only as the 'saviour of its sibling', a role already played by many siblings who donate bone marrow or a kidney.[26] The arguments against the procedure were based on the assumption that such a development would pave the way for 'designer babies', that is, babies born to some parental wish or specification. While Warnock rejects such a 'slippery slope' argument on the grounds that in Britain, the HFEA will always examine each case on its merits, a drift towards genetic selection is now discernible as some European countries prepare to allow sex-selection through IVF for the purpose of 'family balance'.

IVF was initially developed to help infertile couples and this remains its primary function. As is well known, infertility is increasing, for reasons which are only partly understood. Changing patterns of work and lifestyle are clearly a major factor. In the past, women in particular would have had children earlier in life. Now many postpone motherhood until they have established their career, which may well not be until they are in their thirties. By this stage, their fertility will be declining: a recent study has shown that women's *and* men's fertility begins to decline earlier than was previously thought – that of women in their late twenties and that of men in their late thirties. Environmental factors have also been linked, tentatively, with an increase in male infertility.[27] Increasing numbers of people thus turn to IVF, despite its relatively low success rate (currently, there is a 14 per cent chance of success per cycle) and high cost. IVF treatment has had to be strictly rationed in the NHS because of the cost implications, although the National Institute for Clinical Excellence (NICE) has recently recommended that all infertile couples should be offered three free cycles of treatment. Yet despite the cost and difficulty of treatment, at least a million IVF babies have been born since the birth of Louise Brown, the first 'test tube baby', in 1978. In that they are created outside the womb and can survive for four to five days before implantation, such babies can be said to be the products of ectogenesis, with the Petri dish acting as their temporary artificial womb. Moreover, their earliest hours and days of life are not only sustained outside the maternal body, but are open to public view, as dramatised in Rachel Morris's novel *Ella and the Mothers*, in which, after the success of an IVF treatment, one of the characters is summoned to see her fertilised eggs:

She had stood over her test tube and peered down the microscope and seen the embryos divided into eight, like fragments of a blackberry, drawn with pen and ink. Gina had been touched to see that these little bits of her body's essence, which for years had met and mated in darkness and in secrecy, could and would perform for her in public. But even so she had thought that they deserved better. 'Couldn't you at least turn the lights down?' Gina had said to Mr Kalotheou.[28]

In this and other ways, IVF technology thus fractures the 'one flesh' model of pregnancy, separating mother and child in ways that are not only physical but ideological, endowing the embryo with temporary but complete independence from the nurturing womb.

The ever-increasing success in caring for premature babies has a similar effect. In 1987, against all expectations, a baby born at 23 weeks survived, and at 28 weeks a baby is now considered viable if given special care in an incubator.[29] Thus at the beginning and at the end of pregnancy, an 'artificial womb' (Petri dish or incubator) can replace the mother's body: we might say that pregnancy now has its analogues in IVF and incubation.

E. Ann Kaplan has argued that there has been a 'paradigm shift' in relation to childbirth and childcare so that they are 'no longer being viewed as an automatic, natural part of woman's life-cycle'.[30] She connects this shift with (some) women's ability to choose whether or not to be mothers. One might also argue, however, that women are becoming separated from reproduction in the cultural imaginary because the maternal function can, increasingly, be fulfilled ectogenetically.

An alternative treatment for infertility is through xenogenesis (to return to Julian Huxley's term) whereby a surrogate carries a child for another. Surrogacy may depend on IVF to fertilise one of the surrogate's eggs with the sperm of the would-be father or of a donor or, more desirably, an embryo can be created by IVF which is genetically unrelated to the surrogate. Commercial surrogacy is legal in the US, where it has proved both profitable and controversial. It first became widely known with the case of 'Baby M', when a woman who had carried a child for another couple found herself unable to give the baby up after birth. The ensuing legal struggle for the child drew huge media attention, particularly because this was a case in which the surrogate was the biological as well as the surrogate mother.[31] In Britain, surrogacy is not a criminal offence, but a surrogacy contract is not legally binding. Because there is no legal framework for surrogacy it is carried out without medical intervention – in other words, without the assistance of IVF. Thus the surrogate who impregnates herself with the father's sperm or has intercourse with him will always be the biological as well as the birth mother of the resulting child. It is far more likely for a surrogate to find that she is unwilling to give up a child in these circumstances. In view of the precarious nature of such arrangements, Warnock has recently argued in favour of regulation of surrogacy in the UK. Regulation would offer some legal protection for all participants, and would mean that the medical profession could be involved in the process. Thus IVF could be used in a case where, for example, a woman could produce eggs but not sustain a pregnancy: her eggs could be fertilised by her partner's sperm and the surrogate mother would, in theory, be more detached from the process: she would simply be, in Warnock's words, 'lending her womb as a living incubator' (p. 88).

Surrogacy will also play a crucial part in the most controversial treatment yet proposed for infertility: human cloning. Research into animal cloning has been going on for many years, and in 1997 Dolly the sheep was successfully cloned at the Roslin Institute near Edinburgh. The method used was to take a mammary cell from an adult ewe and culture it in the laboratory so that it started to multiply. An egg was then harvested from another ewe, and after its nucleus had been removed, the whole cell from the first ewe was inserted into the egg. After brief exposure to an electric current the egg fused to form a reconstructed embryo. Crucially, however, the embryo was not completely identical, in genetic terms, with the ewe from which the cell material had been taken. In clones formed by nuclear transfer, while the genes come predominantly from the animal from whom the cells are taken, a small amount of DNA is also inherited through the cells lining the egg. The reconstituted embryo is thus not an identical clone, unlike identical twins formed from the natural division of the human embryo.

There is in theory no reason why cloning should not be used in humans, although extreme caution has been urged, not least because Dolly developed signs of premature ageing and arthritis and died in 2003. The cloning process is thus not only difficult technically but currently involves a high degree of risk. Cloning is controversial because many fear that it could be abused by those who are not infertile but simply wish to reproduce themselves genetically. It could also be used to eliminate defects within the population (back to eugenics) or to create large population groups suited for particular tasks (back to *Brave New World*). The use of large-scale cloning thus poses a number of social and scientific problems which are explored in Naomi Mitchison's 1975 novel *Solution Three* (originally entitled *The Clone Mums*). As the sister of J.B.S. Haldane and friend of Julian and Aldous Huxley, Mitchison had a detailed knowledge of evolutionary theory and eugenic thought; in the 1950s she also became a close friend of James Watson, the co-discoverer of DNA, to whom *Solution Three* is dedicated. One effect of this multi-stranded novel is, through inversion, to offer a deft and incisive critique of the racism and homophobia which (still) structures Western society. The fictional world of *Solution Three* has been drastically reorganised after a period of over-population and inter-racial 'aggressions'. Population is now rigorously controlled, and it has been agreed that the world should be repopulated only with clones of 'Him' and 'Her', a black American man and a white woman from the Shetlands who, in their struggles for world peace and justice, are considered types of the ideal human being. Heterosexual reproduction is thus more or less outlawed, the only group which still practises it being the Professorials. Their lifestyle is stigma-tised as deviant and their relationships have to be hidden; for everyone else, sexual desire is expressed through same-sex relationships.

Through parallel plots linked through the characterisation of a 'deviant' plant geneticist, the novel highlights the dangers of genetic engineering and cloning. Miryam is sent out to Central Asia to monitor wheat crops threatened by disease. These crops have been carefully bred to give the highest possible yield, but it is precisely this careful breeding which has removed genes offering protection against certain viruses and bacteria. Moreover, a mutation may have occurred which has made the crops vulnerable to a particular infection. Miryam realises that she must track down older, discarded strains of wheat (if any have survived) in order to rebuild the wheat programme with a variety that can withstand the new threat. And, the novel suggests, as with wheat, so with human beings. Darwinian theory assumes that evolution depends on diversity in the gene pool. Natural selection ensures that those best adapted to the environment survive and repro-duce (often benefiting from a small but favourable genetic mutation). However, if the environment suddenly changes, individuals with a very different genetic make-up will be required for species survival. If the human gene pool has been severely restricted, as in the mass cloning experiment in *Solution Three*, the human race will be without the genetic resources needed for adaptation and survival. It is Mutumba, the controller of the world of *Solution Three*, who makes the connection between the fate of the wheat and the potential fate of the human race, in a conversation about the need for a 'wheat pool':

'A wheat pool,' said Mutumba. 'Okay. But are we sure, Jussie, are we quite sure, that we shall never need to get ourselves a human gene pool? And as varied as it comes? Now, Jussie, I'm asking you to think in these terms: a kind of excellence which exactly fitted a certain epoch might, soon or late, need certain alterations. The wheat was the best of its species: something went wrong. Now we have to start again ... back crossing to something we thought we'd finished with. Yes?'

'Mutumba, you are not saying you have doubts about – about the Clones?'[32]

Mitchison's argument in *Solution Three* is not only that cloning-as-replication is not desirable for the long-term future of the race, but that it is not, strictly speaking, possible because of the influence of the environment on the developing child before as well as after birth. In making the latter point she challenges the view of surrogacy as a kind of rental arrangement, involving no emotional or physical exchanges between mother and unborn child. This issue is explored through the character of Lilac, one of the 'clone mums' who is deviant in a different sense from Miryam. Lilac does not harbour heterosexual desires, but feels a passionate love for her clone baby. She feels, heretically, that the baby has not simply been lent to her but is in some sense part of her, and she tries to defer the time when he will be taken from her for 'strengthening' (conditioning). However, when her delaying tactics have been discovered, she is not punished but offered work researching the bond between surrogate and child. It appears that although the 'clone mums' have had their cell nucleus removed, the children they carry will be affected by the nature of the maternal environment and by the 'interchange of fluids between the foetus and its host' (p. 99). The child may be affected by hormones circulating through the placenta and, according to Mutumba, it might even be that some genetic information comes to the foetus from the surrogate's maternal cytoplasm.[33] Mitchison situates Mutumba's interest in this question firmly in the context of her broader concerns about species variation. However, by focusing too on Lilac's subjective experiences, Mitchison highlights the implications of such a reinterpretation of surrogacy for the individual mother. For if it were accepted that the surrogate has a significant input into and influence on the development of a child, the relationship between surrogate and child would have to be refigured in social, ethical and legal terms.

Doris Lessing's novel *The Fifth Child* (1988) explores the reverse of the situation in *Solution Three*. Whereas in Mitchison's novel reproduction has been so constrained that society has to go in deliberate search of earlier genetic material, in Lessing's text such material erupts unpre-dictably and damagingly into the contemporary world. Almost from the moment of his conception, the eponymous fifth child of a conven-tional middle-class couple is apprehended as a hostile presence. During her pregnancy his mother, Harriett, claims that the foetus is poisoning her: the foetal movements are so violent and painful that she has to walk endlessly to distract herself or use sedatives to calm the baby down. As the pregnancy progresses, she begins to think of it in terms of monstrosity or cross-species breeding:

> Phantoms and chimeras inhabited her brain. She would think, When the scientists make experiments, welding two kinds of animal together, of different sizes, then I suppose this is what the poor mother feels. She imagined pathetic botched creatures, horribly real to her, the products of a Great Dane or a borzoi with a little spaniel; a lion and a dog; a great cart horse and a little donkey; a tiger and a goat. Sometimes she believed hooves were cutting her tender inside flesh, sometimes claws.[34]

Lessing here invokes two discourses: one of the imaginative tradition of the chimerical or monstrous (of beings which cannot exist in nature); the other of experimental science, which has not only undertaken cross-breeding between animal species but has created hybrids of human and animal tissues.[35] However, after the birth of the child, another interpretive framework comes into play. Ben's physical appearance is initially described in simian terms: 'He did not look like a baby at all. He had a heavy-shouldered hunched look, as if he were crouching there as he lay. His forehead sloped from his eyes to his crown ... His hands were thick and heavy' (p. 60). Seeing him with other children in the institution in which he is placed for a while, Harriett contemplates the ways in which the human genetic template can falter or mutate and eventually comes to the conclusion that Ben is an anachronism, an evolutionary 'throwback':

> She felt she was looking, through him, at a race that reached its apex thousands and thousands of years before humanity, whatever that meant, took this stage. Did Ben's people live in caves under-ground while the ice age ground overhead ...? Did his people rape the females of humanity's forebears? Thus making new races, which had flourished and departed, but perhaps had left their seeds in the human matrix, here and there, to appear again, as Ben had? (p. 156)

Lessing thus draws on the language of evolutionary theory and genetics as an explanatory framework for monstrosity. The novel invites comparison with *Frankenstein* in some ways – for example, Ben resembles Frankenstein's monster in his sallow, waxy, *unhealthy* appearance. He is not, however, a laboratory creation, and is closely identified with his biological mother in the eyes of others. Harriett thus becomes, in time-honoured fashion, a maternal scapegoat: 'Even David [her husband], she believed, condemned her. She said to him, "I suppose in the old times, in primitive societies, this was how they treated a woman who'd given birth to a freak. As if it was her fault. But we are supposed to be civilized!"' (p. 74). Yet Harriett feels no close link with her son: she too finds him alien and impenetrable. The text thus begins to problematise the idea of a 'natural' bond inhering in biological motherhood. In positing a rogue gene or genetic throwback, Lessing draws attention to the fact that genetic material can be suppressed for long periods and then 'switched on' in specific circumstances. In other words, the genetic material we inherit from our parents may go back generations and, more crucially, may not be 'expressed' in them. Through the extreme case of Ben, Lessing's text thus begins to demystify biological/genetic motherhood, emphasising the fact that it can involve discontinuity and difference as well as continuity and likeness.

Reproductive choices

Over the last three decades, family structures have changed markedly in Britain, in part because women have gained more financial independence as they have moved into the workplace in greater numbers, in part because the contraceptive pill has given them greater sexual freedom and reproductive control. Moreover, as Anthony Giddens has argued in *The Transformation of Intimacy*, now that conception can be artificially prevented and artificially produced, sex has become largely divorced from reproduction and has turned into sexuality, something far more malleable and open to change. The term Giddens coins for this is 'plastic sexuality', that is, sex severed from 'its age-old integration with reproduction, kinship and the generations'.[36] According to Giddens, when sex and reproduction do now coincide, it is more often than not in the context of the 'confluent love' which, he argues, is replacing the 'romantic love complex' grounded in a belief in love for life. The 'separating and divorcing' society of today is thus, he contends, 'an effect of the emergence of confluent love rather than its cause'. However, an issue Giddens does not address is that in an era of 'plastic sexuality' and confluent love, reproduction becomes a complex and risky undertaking. In cases where a relationship breaks down and there are children, in the vast majority of cases it is the mother who will become the single parent. This usually has severe financial implications for them, as the mother is unlikely to have been the primary earner.

In their study 'Becoming a Single Mother', Richard Berthoud, Stephen McKay and Karen Rowlingson have analysed in detail the rise in the numbers of lone-parent families in Britain.[37] In 1971 there were about 570,000 lone parents; by 1995 there were more than 1.5 million. As they point out, there are several different types of lone-parent family, although in nine cases out of ten such families are headed by the mother. Until the 1990s the largest group consisted of women who had children while married and who subsequently separated and divorced (according to the pattern described by Giddens). A small and shrinking number of lone-parent families are headed by widows. The most rapidly growing group is of women who have never married prior to motherhood: such women outnumbered divorced lone mothers for the first time in 1991. By 1994, one in twelve of all families with dependent children was headed by a never-married mother. In this study, the authors make a further distinction between lone mothers who have never married but have lived with the father of their child/ren ('separated lone mothers'), and those who have never married or cohabited with the father ('single mothers'). The latter group has increased over the last thirty years, and such women now remain single for longer after the birth of a child. While both 'separated lone mothers' and 'single mothers' often come from disadvantaged backgrounds (using a measure of social class based on the woman's father's occupation), this is by no means always the case, and the authors of the study have identified changing social attitudes which are affecting women of all classes. Their research supports the view that single motherhood is no longer considered shameful but has become an acceptable, if not always a desirable, condition. One respondent in the interviews undertaken for the study described her parents' reaction to her pregnancy in these terms: 'I had their full support, what I wanted. If I wanted to carry on through the pregnancy, it was perfectly fine ... I was under no pressure at all' (p. 370). Such support enabled the women who were interviewed to reject the options of 'shotgun weddings', abortion and adoption which might previously have been forced on them. Many women expressed opposition to abortion as a matter of principle, while adoption was widely rejected and seen as incompatible with a female caring identity (p. 371). 'Choices' are, of course, determined or constrained by ideological as well as by practical contexts: from the evidence of this study, it seems that single motherhood is now more socially acceptable than abortion or adoption.

One group of single mothers who have attracted a good deal of attention are professional women who decide to have a child without having a male (or female) partner. Such a decision may be linked with fear of the ticking of the biological clock, a subject which has received massive media coverage and which has been associated with the catchphrase 'babyhunger'.[38] Perhaps in consequence, the single professional mother now has a sub-genre to herself, pregnant chick lit. Books such as Maeve Haran's *All That She Wants* (1998) and Jane Green's *Babyville* (2002) offer interestingly partial explorations of single motherhood. The heroine of *All That She Wants* is the 'flame-haired' Francesca, a career woman in her thirties who decides to become pregnant despite the fact that she has no male partner.[39] As in other texts in this sub-genre, fear of infertility hovers in the background: Francesca is not infertile herself, but visits a clinic in her capacity as a journalist and subsequently becomes involved with its director, Laurence. She also has a brief affair with another man, so that when she discovers she is pregnant she has no means of telling which is the father. However, after various complications, she discovers that the biological father is the man she loves, and that he wants to marry her. Pregnancy is thus reunited with romantic love and genetic inheritance realigned with parenthood. This feel-good ending enables Haran (and her readers) to sidestep the challenges set up earlier in the novel. Francesca avoids the financial hardship of single motherhood and the difficulties of uncertain paternity or of bringing up a child with a man who is not the biological father. The importance of biological ties and biological fitness for reproduction is strongly emphasised through the characterisation of Francesca's lovers. Jack is a 'natural' father, able to soothe a crying baby by holding it against his rough tweed jacket: he has also been an effective single parent for his son. Laurence, in contrast, has been emotionally scarred by the fact that he is adopted and also turns out to be infertile. So strong is the text's bias in favour of 'the natural' that it almost seems that his adoption and his infertility are in some sense causally linked.

Babyville similarly forecloses many of the difficulties associated with single motherhood.[40] The main focus is on Maeve, a single woman (again working in the media) who becomes pregnant after a one-night stand. Though she initially plans to have an abortion, she decides to go ahead with the pregnancy, with the friendly support of the father. Opportunely, she and the father fall in love before the birth, so that again romantic love and pregnancy coincide and Maeve is spared the financial and emotional embarrassments of single motherhood. While this novel arguably breaks new ground in its treatment of sex in pregnancy, it generally endorses deeply conventional attitudes to reproduction.

By contrast, Rachel Morris's *Ella and the Mothers* contests such attitudes, especially in relation to the biological link between parent and child. The plot is relatively easy to summarise. Ella's mother, Madeleine Kingdom, has been left by her husband while they are undergoing a course of fertility treatment. She decides to continue with the process, but using donor sperm. The plot turns on an IVF mix-up and the pursuit and eventual kidnap of Ella by Gina, who is convinced that she is Ella's biological mother. It transpires (unknown to Madeleine) that neither woman is the mother: an embryo from another couple has been implanted in Madeleine's womb. Through plot and characterisation, this novel interrogates the ideology of biological motherhood, whereby the genetic link between mother and child is not only construed as natural but is naturalised, and other forms of motherhood devalued. Through the character of Gina in particular, Morris calls attention to the way in which biological motherhood has become mythologised. When she discovers that Ella might be her child, Gina tells herself that she is the 'real' mother, and goes on to recall a scrap of popular mythology from the 'Baby M' surrogacy case: 'She'd once heard of a surrogate baby whose adopted parents couldn't stop it crying, and whom only the real mother could soothe, because the biological tie was that important.'[41] Here, the language of the fairy tale ('the real mother') highlights the element of fantasy and wish-fulfilment involved in the notion of the 'blood tie'. By contrast, when Madeleine thinks about the fact that Ella might not be hers, she finds that 'what was interesting was that this idea, which was so enormous, in reality changed nothing ... because this equally was true, that she didn't care where Ella came from, she could have come from the moon for all that it mattered. All that she could feel was that she had loved and nurtured and toiled for this child and now they were linked together indissolubly' (p. 138). Like *The Fifth Child*, the novel thus questions the inviolability of the genetic tie. Genetic motherhood does not guarantee sameness or compatibility (for genes can skip generations, and the reassortment of genes which accompanies the division of egg and sperm provides further grounds for difference). It is not genes, but the work of 'loving, nurturing and toiling' which create the 'indissoluble tie' of motherhood. The choice of the word 'toil' is significant: the novel does not shrink from registering the effort required to bring up a child alone, combining a full-time job and domestic responsibilities (in the early years, Madeleine also has to have daytime child-care, which is a significant drain on her income).

Despite the hardships she encounters after Ella's birth, Madeleine is fortunate in that she can afford private fertility treatment, even without her husband's income. IVF is not usually offered to single mothers or lesbian couples on the NHS (although as the fertility specialist Lord Winston has acknowledged, doctors find it difficult to provide rational reasons for this form of selection, which may change with the new NICE guidelines on fertility treatment).[42] Madeleine's pregnancy can thus be seen as something of a consumer choice, and this raises the broader question of the commodification of pregnancy in a technologically sophisticated consumer society.

In an article addressing this issue, Janelle S. Taylor has argued that the feminist analogy posited in the 1980s between reproduction and industrial production remains a compelling one.[43] Indeed, in an era of pre-natal diagnostic tests and other new reproductive technologies, the language of mass production can seem still more pertinent: 'Doctors have come to be positioned as "managers" relative to reproduction, fetuses appear as valuable "products", and women are like reproductive "workers"' (pp. 392–3), However, Taylor goes on to argue that we can enrich our understanding of contemporary pregnancy by interpreting it in terms of consumption as well as production. Her argument is based on ethnographic research carried out in an obstetrics clinic in Chicago, which led her to conclude that 'the same transformations that have positioned women as "workers" relative to reproduction have also offered up to them the pleasures of reproduction construed as consumption' (p. 397). In a sense, this could be read as a reworking of Iris Young's point that the experience of pregnancy undoes the opposition between subject and object, so that the pregnant body 'attends positively to itself at the same time that it enacts its projects'.[44] However, Taylor's argument that the pregnant woman produces what she consumes (the foetus as prospective child) is located in a more specific social and cultural context.

In August 1991, Annie Leibewitz's *Vanity Fair* cover image of a naked and heavily pregnant Demi Moore inaugurated an era in which the pregnant body began to be construed in terms of glamour and desirability.[45]

Leibewitz's portrait constructed Moore as both desirable (a glamorous object of the gaze) and desirous (clasping her pregnant belly 'exactly as she might a bulging shopping bag', as Matthews and Wexler put it).[46] Numerous images of 'pregnant icons' have followed which invest pregnancy with (competing) consuming passions. The pregnant woman is invited both to construct herself as eroticised object, with appropriate clothing and accessories, and to construct her foetus as the end and object of her pregnancy (provided, again, with appropriate clothing and accessories bought well in advance of the birth). At the same time, as Taylor points out, new reproductive technologies have made it possible for various 'consumer choices' to be made in relation to pregnancy. Women can opt for technocratic or holistic styles of pre-natal care, they can negotiate a convenient date for delivery and, of course, they can access a number of forms of assisted conception.

The commodification of (some aspects of) pregnancy can be linked with a broader shift in European and American economies from material culture to consumer culture. As Celia Lury puts it, this can be characterised in terms of an intensified deployment of consumer goods 'as if they were works of art, images or signs and as part of the self-conscious creation of lifestyle'.[47] This shift has affected almost all aspects of life and accounts, for example, for the proliferation of consumer goods and services now available as accoutrements of pregnancy (clothes, dedicated foods, exercise classes, and so on).

A further factor in the commodification of pregnancy is an increasing readiness on the part of individual women and men to invest (in all senses) in a child. It has been argued that in a 'separating and divorcing society', the parent/child bond has come to seem more significant and more permanent than the marital/sexual bond.[48] Thus, for both women and men, pregnancy represents an extremely significant life-event, which they want to mark as a rite of passage: hence the importation into this country of the American 'baby shower', at which gifts are presented for the coming child. (It is surely significant in this respect that men are now happy to describe themselves as 'being pregnant', metaphorically incorporating themselves into a process previously marked off as feminine.) In Britain, a final crucial factor is the introduction of the market economy into areas previously considered the responsibility of the state. 'Internal markets' have been created in the NHS and patients are now encouraged to see themselves as 'consumers' of medical care and encouraged to consider private options if the NHS is unable to 'deliver' the desired goods.

Yet such 'choices' are only available to the well-off. As Zygmunt Bauman has pointed out, 'behind the ostensible equality of chances the market promotes and advertises hides the practical inequality of consumers – that is, the sharply differentiated degrees of practical freedom of choice'.[49] Over the last three decades, income inequality in Britain has grown more rapidly than in any other industrialised country. Between 1979 and 1995, average incomes grew by 40 per cent, but the incomes of the richest 10 per cent grew by over 60 per cent, while those of the poorest 10 per cent grew by 10 per cent. In 1995, 18 per cent of the population had incomes below half the contemporary average, a three-fold increase on the figure in 1977.[50] A significant and growing proportion of the population are thus living below the poverty line and are entirely dependent on state support and benefits. For those on low incomes, or on no income, the consumer choices considered above do not exist. The inability to buy consumer goods targeted at pregnant women may not seem very significant, but it contributes to a pervasive sense of failure and social exclusion. Higher up the scale, lack of access to exercise classes or a healthy diet may impact adversely on the outcome of the pregnancy (and on the life-chances of the child). It scarcely needs to be added that the difficulty many couples have experienced in gaining access to free fertility treatment has created an enormous amount of disstress and unhappiness. Thus, while in absolute terms the health of pregnant women and of their foetuses has improved beyond all recognition since the Second World War, the inequalities between pregnant women remain as great, and may have become even greater. Pregnancy in Britain thus remains an extremely diverse, and class-specific, experience.

Notes

Introduction

1. See the Introduction to Malcolm Elwin, *The Noels and the Milbankes: Their Letters for Twenty-Five Years, 1767–1792* (London: Macdonald, 1967) for details of Judith Milbanke's marriage. Subsequent references to this source are incorporated into the text.
2. A stoppage was an obstruction of the womb, which could be confused with pregnancy, as could 'moles' and 'false conceptions'.
3. Exactly a year after Annabella married Byron in 1815, she demanded a separation and began to assemble a mass of documents relating to her marriage. Having got into the habit of documentation and preservation, she also kept all the letters handed down to her by her mother, Judith Milbanke.
4. Rachel Cusk, *A Life's Work: On Becoming a Mother* (London: Fourth Estate, 2001), p. 23. Subsequent references are incorporated into the text.
5. Jill L. Matus, *Unstable Bodies: Victorian Representations of Sexuality and Maternity* (Manchester and New York: Manchester University Press, 1995), p. 6.
6. Evelyn Fox Keller, *The Century of the Gene* (Cambridge, Mass. and London: Harvard University Press, 2000), p. 139.
7. E. Ann Kaplan, *Motherhood and Representation: The Mother in Popular Culture and Melodrama* (London: Routledge, 1992), p. 19.
8. Ann Oakley, *The Captured Womb: A History of the Medical Care of Pregnant Women* (Oxford: Blackwell, 1984), p. 14. In relation to women's anxiety about death in childbirth (as opposed to anxiety about foetal health), Irvine Loudon has argued convincingly against the 'wide-eyed open-mouthed view of childbirth in the past that is shared by some historians', who paint a picture of 'terrified women dying in childbirth like flies'. As he points out, risk is always relative, and the risk of dying in childbirth is perceived at any given time in the context of other risks to women of childbearing age. Thus, in 1890, when maternal mortality was at its highest at any point in history, it still accounted for only 8.8 per cent of deaths from all causes among women aged 15–44. See Irvine Loudon, *Death in Childbirth: An International Study of Maternal Care and Maternal Mortality 1800–1950* (Oxford: Clarendon Press, 1992), pp. 162–3.
9. Royal Commission on Population, *Report* (London: HMSO, 1949), p. 134.
10. See Leonore Davidoff and Catherine Hall, *Family Fortunes: Men and Women of the English Middle Class, 1780–1850* (London: The University of Chicago Press, 1987), pp. 205–6.
11. The current legal position in England, Scotland and Wales is that a woman has the right to abortion (in the first twenty-four weeks of pregnancy) when it is needed for the sake of her health. She can obtain an abortion only if

she can find two doctors willing to say that her health requires it. However, the law construes 'women's health' very broadly, to include social as well as strictly medical considerations. In Northern Ireland, threats to a woman's health are understood far more narrowly.

12. See Thomas Malthus, *An Essay on the Principle of Population as It Affects the Future Improvement of Society, With Remarks on the Speculations of Mr Godwin, M. Condorcet, And Other Writers* (London: J. Johnson, 1798).
13. See, for example, G.F. McCleary, *Race Suicide?* (London: George Allen and Unwin, 1945), p. 27, for a discussion of the impact of contraceptive knowledge in the nineteenth century.
14. William Smellie, *A Treatise on the Theory and Practice of Midwifery* (London: D. Wilson, 1752), Vol. 1, p. 280.
15. J.W. Ballantyne, 'A Plea for a Pro-Maternity Hospital', *British Medical Journal* (6 April 1901), p. 815. For concerns about a fall in the birth rate, see, for example, C.W. Saleeby, *Woman and Womanhood: A Search for Principles* (London: William Heinemann, 1912).
16. Puerperal fever was the single most important cause of maternal mortality until the mid-twentieth century. The fact that it was spread by contagion was known in the mid-nineteenth century, and obstetricians such as James Simpson argued for what was then known as 'antisepsis', i.e. general cleanliness on the part of doctors and midwives, in order to cut down the risk of disease. In the late 1860s Lister's use of carbolic acid ushered in antiseptic procedures as we now know them, but puerperal fever rates remained relatively high. It was not until the early 1940s, with the use of sulphonamides and then penicillin, that the mortality rate from infected cases fell dramatically. See *The Queen Charlotte's Textbook of Obstetrics*, eighth edition, ed. G.F. Gibberd et al. (London: J. and A. Churchill, 1952), p. 347, for a discussion of this.
17. See Evelyn M. Bunting (ed.), *A School for Mothers* (London: Horace Marshall & Son, 1907), p. 9.
18. J.W. Ballantyne, *Expectant Motherhood: Its Supervision and Hygiene* (London, New York, Toronto and Melbourne: Cassell, 1914), p. 53.
19. John Grigg, *Advice to the Female Sex in General, Particularly those in a State of Pregnancy and Lying-in: The Complaints incident to their respective Situations are specified, and Treatment recommended, Agreeable to Modern Practice* (Bath: S. Hazard, 1789), p. 7; Martha Mears, *The Midwife's Candid Advice to the Fair Sex: or the Pupil of Nature*, A New Edition (London: Crosby and Co. and R. Faulder, 1805), p. 4.
20. Margery Spring Rice, *Working-class Wives: Their Health and Conditions*, with an Introduction by Dame Janet Campbell (Harmondsworth: Penguin Books, 1939), pp. 157–8.
21. See David J.P. Barker, 'The Malnourished Baby and Infant' in *Type 2 Diabetes: The Thrifty Phenotype, British Medical Bulletin*, ed. David J.P. Barker, Vol. 60 (2001), pp. 69–88.
22. See *Understanding Pregnancy*, published in association with the British Medical Association (Family Doctor Publications: Poole, 2002), p. 15.
23. W.F. Montgomery, *An Exposition of the Signs and Symptoms of Pregnancy, the Period of Human Gestation, and the Signs of Delivery* (London: Sherwood, Gilbert, & Piper, 1837), p. 32.

24. See S.L. Barron, 'Introduction', in S.L. Barron and D.F. Roberts (eds), *Issues in Fetal Medicine: Proceedings of the Twenty-Ninth Annual Symposium of the Galton Institute, London 1992* (Basingstoke: Macmillan, in association with The Galton Institute, 1995) for a discussion of issues arising in relation to the 'foetal patient'.

25. For the most influential discussion of the medicalisation of the body, see Michel Foucault, *The Birth of the Clinic*, trans. Alan Sheridan (London: Routledge, 1997).

26. See Grigg, *Advice to the Female Sex in General*; Alexander Hamilton, *A Treatise of Midwifery Comprehending the Management of Female Complaints, and the Treatment of Children in Early Infancy* (London: J. Murray and Edinburgh: Dickson, Creech and Elliot, 1781), Mears, *The Midwife's Candid Advice*; and Elizabeth Nihell, *A Treatise on the Art of Midwifery* (London: A. Morley, 1760).

27. W.O. Priestley and Horatio R. Storer (eds), *The Obstetric Memoirs and Contributions of James Y. Simpson, Professor of Midwifery in the University of Edinburgh* (Edinburgh: Adam and Charles Black, 1854), Vol. 11, pp. 619 and 701.

28. Herbert Spencer, *The Study of Sociology*, seventeenth edition (London: Kegan Paul, Trench, Trubner & Co., Ltd., 1894), p. 373.

29. Kelly Oliver (ed.), *The Portable Kristeva* (New York and Chichester: Columbia University Press, 1997), p. 301.

30. Sigmund Freud, *On Metapsychology*, Pelican Freud Library 11 (Harmondsworth: Pelican Books, 1984), pp. 364–5.

31. See Jacques Lacan, 'The Mirror Stage as Formative of the Function of the I as Revealed in Psychoanalytic Experience', in *Ecrits: A Selection*, trans. Alan Sheridan (London: Tavistock, 1977); Didier Anzieu, *The Skin Ego: A Psychoanalytic Approach to the Self*, trans. Chris Turner (New Haven: Yale University Press, 1989).

32. Mary Douglas, *Purity and Danger: An Analysis of Concepts of Pollution and Taboo* (Harmondsworth: Pelican Books, 1970)

33. William Smellie, *Anatomical Tables with Explanations and an Abridgement of the Practice of Midwifery, with a view to illustrate A Treatise on that Subject and Collection of Cases* (Edinburgh: William Creech, 1754); William Hunter, *Anatomia Uteri Humani Gravidi: Tabulis Illustrata* (Birmingham; John Baskerville, 1774); William Smellie, *A Treatise on the Theory and Practice of Midwifery*, 3 vols. (London: D. Wilson, 1752–64); Alexander Hamilton, *A Treatise of Midwifery Comprehending the Management of Female Complaints, and the Treatment of Children in Early Infancy ...Divested of Technical Terms and Abstruse Theories* (London: J. Murray; Edinburgh: Dickson, Creech and Elliot, 1781); Thomas Denman, *An Introduction to the Practice of Midwifery* (London: J. Johnson, 1788). In the 'Preface' to the first volume of his treatise on midwifery, Smellie recorded that he had taught over 900 pupils, exclusive of female students. Hunter's anatomical lectures were also extremely well attended.

34. Erasmus Darwin, *Zoonomia: Or, The Laws of Organic Life* (London: J. Johnson, 1794), Preface, pp. 1–2.

35. Loudon, *Death in Childbirth*, p. 171.

Chapter 1

1. See Jean Donnison, *Midwives and Medical Men: A History of Inter-Professional Rivalries and Women's Rights* (London: Heinemann, 1977); Hilary Marland (ed.), *The Art of Midwifery: Early Modern Midwives in Europe* (London: Routledge, 1993); O. Moscucci, *The Science of Woman: Gynaecology and Gender in England, 1800–1929* (Cambridge: Cambridge University Press, 1990); and Adrian Wilson, *The Making of Man-Midwifery* (Cambridge, Mass.: Harvard University Press, 1995).

2. Elizabeth Nihell, *A Treatise on the Art of Midwifery. Setting forth various abuses therein, especially as to the practice with instruments: the whole serving to put all rational inquirers in a fair way of very safely forming their own judgment upon the question; what it is best to employ, in cases of pregnancy and lying-in, a man-midwife or, a midwife* (London, A. Morley, 1760), p. 232. Subsequent references are incorporated into the text.

3. Anonymous line engraving from 1773, published by S. Hooper, entitled 'The man-midwife, or female delicacy after marriage: addressed to husbands'. Wellcome Trust Medical Picture Library.

4. Alexander Hamilton, *A Treatise of Midwifery Comprehending the Management of Female Complaints, and the Treatment of Children in Early Infancy ...Divested of Technical Terms and Abstruse Theories* (London: J. Murray; Edinburgh: Dickson, Creech and Elliot, 1781), p. 109. Subsequent references are incorporated into the text.

5. Tobias Smollett, quoted in Philip K. Wilson (ed.), *Childbirth: Changing Ideas and Practices in Britain and America 1600 to the Present* (New York and London: Garland Publishing, 1996), Vol. 2, pp. 47–8.

6. Midwives continued to attend poorer women in the late eighteenth and nineteenth centuries, and a considerable number had some training. However, we have no accurate information about the number of women who engaged midwives (as opposed to male practitioners), nor about the numbers who were attended by friends or family members. See Irvine Loudon, *Death in Childbirth: An International Study of Maternal Care and Maternal Mortality 1800–1950* (Oxford: Clarendon Press, 1992), chapter 11, for a discussion of this. Loudon has suggested elsewhere that by the 1790s, 'something between a third and a half of all deliveries in England were attended by medical practitioners'. See Irvine Loudon (ed.), *Western Medicine: An Illustrated History* (Oxford: Oxford University Press, 1997), p. 209.

7. This was just one upward route among many in the unstable world of late eighteenth-century medicine, in which surgeon-apothecaries were jockeying for territory and status. Smith's novel *The Young Philosopher* alludes to the uncertain professional standing of physicians: the narrator describes medicine as 'that noble profession, which is never enough respected, but which, when attentively studied and conscientiously followed, is the most beneficial of any to the human race' (1: 84)

8. William Hunter, 'On the Uncertainty of the Signs of Murder in the Case of Bastard Children' (London: J. Callow, 1812), p. 6. Paper read to the Medical Society, 14 July 1783. Subsequent references are incorporated into the text.

9. Laënnec invented the stethoscope in 1819. When it was used by his pupil Kergaradec to listen to the 'splashing' of the foetus *in utero*, the foetal heartbeat was picked up for the first time. See E.T.H. Laënnec, *Treatise on Mediate Auscultation and Diseases of the Lung and Heart*, trans. J. Forbes, second edition, 1827.

10. Thomas Denman, *An Introduction to the Practice of Midwifery* (London: J. Johnson, 1788), p. 337. Subsequent references are incorporated into the text.

11. See John Grigg, *Advice to the Female Sex in General, Particularly those in a State of Pregnancy and Lying-in* (Bath: S. Hazard, 1789), p. 80. Subsequent references are incorporated into the text.

12. Joanna Southcott, *Memoirs of the Life and Mission of Joanna Southcott, interspersed with Authentic Anecdotes and elucidated by Interesting Documents including the Progress of her Pregnancy detailed by herself together with the Opinions of Drs Reece and Sims to which is added a Sketch of the Rev. W. Tozer, M.J.S. embellished with a Striking Likeness of the Prophetress* (London: M. Jones, 1814), p. 24. Subsequent references are incorporated into the text.

13. W.F. Montgomery, *An Exposition of the Signs and Symptoms of Pregnancy, the Period of Human Gestation, and the Signs of Delivery* (London: Sherwood, Gilbert, & Piper, 1837), p. 85. Subsequent references are incorporated into the text.

14. Martha Mears, *The Midwife's Candid Advice to the Fair Sex; or the Pupil of Nature*, new edition (London: Crosby and Co. and R. Faulder, 1805), pp. 5–6, emphasis added. Subsequent references are incorporated into the text.

15. Albrecht von Haller had shown that irritability (contractility) was a property inherent in all muscular fibres, whereas sensibility was the exclusive attribute of nervous fibres, which responded to painful stimuli.

16. My reading of Mears has a somewhat different emphasis from that of Amanda Gilroy. In her essay '"Candid Advice to the Fair Sex": or, the Politics of Maternity in Late Eighteenth-century Britain', Gilroy argues that Mears 'depletes maternal agency' and 'represents not just female bodies in need of restraint but minds oppressed'. See Avril Horner and Angela Keane (eds), *Body Matters: Feminism, Textuality, Corporeality* (Manchester: Manchester University Press, 2000), p. 26.

17. See Philip K. Wilson, '"Out of Sight, Out of Mind?": The Daniel Turner-James Blondel Dispute over the Power of the Maternal Imagination', in Philip K. Wilson (ed.), *Childbirth* (New York and London: Garland Publishing, 1996), Vol. 3, pp. 361–83.

18. William Smellie, *A Treatise on the Theory and Practice of Midwifery* (London: D. Wilson and T. Durham, 1754), Vol. 2, pp. 209–10. Subsequent references are incorporated into the text.

19. Erasmus Darwin, *Zoonomia: Or, The Laws of Organic Life* (London: J. Johnson, 1794), Vol. 2, p. 520. Subsequent references will be incorporated into the text.

20. With reference to the paternal imagination, Darwin unblushingly offers the following anecdote to explain the birth of children who resemble neither parent. An acquaintance of his had a very dark-eyed child, although both parents were fair. This friend told him that 'when his lady lay in of her third child, he became attached to a daughter of one of his inferior tenants,

and offered her a bribe for her favours in vain; and afterwards a greater
bribe, and was equally unsuccessful; that the form of this girl dwelt much
in his mind for some weeks, and that the next child, which was the dark-
ey'd young lady above mentioned, was exceedingly like, in both features
and colour, to the young woman who refused his addresses' (*Zoonomia*,
Vol. 2, pp. 523–4).

21. Mary Wollstonecraft, *Political Writings* (Oxford: Oxford World's Classics,
1994), p. 73.
22. Ralph M. Wardle (ed.), *Collected Letters of Mary Wollstonecraft* (Ithaca, NY
and London: Cornell University Press, 1979), p. 243 (letter of 6 January
1784). Subsequent references are incorporated into the text.
23. Janet Todd (ed.), Mary Wollstonecraft, *Mary* and *Maria*; Mary Shelley,
Matilda (Harmondsworth: Penguin, 1991), p. 126. Subsequent references are
incorporated into the text.
24. Amelia Opie, *Adeline Mowbray* (1805) (Oxford: Oxford World's Classics,
1999), p. 131. Subsequent references are incorporated into the text.
25. See especially Mary Hays, *The Victim of Prejudice* (1799), ed. Eleanor Ty
(Ontario, New York and Cardiff; Broadview Press, 1994); and Charlotte
Smith, *Montalbert* (1795) and *The Young Philosopher* (1798). In all these
novels the stories of daughters repeat (to some degree) the stories of
mothers: names are also repeated or closely echoed.
26. Loraine Fletcher, *Charlotte Smith: A Critical Biography* (Basingstoke: Palgrave,
1998), pp. 279–80. There is a degree of conscious intertextual referencing in
this cluster of novels fictionalising Wollstonecraft's life. Thus, in *Adeline
Mowbray*, the name Opie gives her Godwin figure (Glenmurray) is very
similar to that Smith gives the Tom Paine figure (Glenmorris) in *The Young
Philosopher*.
27. Charlotte Smith, *The Young Philosopher: A Novel*, 4 vols (London: T. Cadeli,
Jun. and W. Davies, 1798), Vol. 1, pp. 106–7. Subsequent references are
incorporated into the text.
28. William Buchan, *Domestic Medicine or, a Treatise on the Prevention and Cure of
Diseases by Regimen and Simple Medicines*, second edition (London:
W. Strachan, and T.Cadell; Edinburgh: A. Kincaid & W. Creech, and
J. Balfour, 1772), p. 140. Subsequent references are incorporated into the
text. *Domestic Medicine* was first published in 1769, the first edition being
part-authored by William Smellie, who revised and to some extent rewrote
Buchan's original manuscript. New editions, reprints and pirated versions
appeared every few years in Britain until 1846. For a discussion of the
success of Buchan's work, see C.J. Lawrence, 'William Buchan: Medicine
Laid Open', in *Medical History*, Vol. 19 (1975), pp. 20–35.
29. The text has a personal resonance. Smith's favourite daughter, Augusta,
died in 1795, probably of tuberculosis exacerbated by a pregnancy for
which she had been attended by Denman. See Fletcher, *Charlotte Smith*,
p. 227.
30. Jane Austen, *Sense and Sensibility*, ed. Mary Lascelles (London: Dent, 1967),
pp. 135–6. Subsequent references are incorporated into the text.
31. Maud Ellmann, *The Hunger Artists: Starving, Writing and Imprisonment*
(London: Virago, 1993), p. 44.

32. Adam Smith, *An Inquiry into the Nature and Causes of the Wealth of Nations*, ed. R.H. Campbell, A.S. Skinner and W.B. Todd (Oxford: Clarendon Press, 1976), Vol. 1, pp. 96–7.

33. See Judith Schneid Lewis, *In the Family Way: Childbearing in the British Aristocracy, 1760–1860* (New Brunswick: Rutgers University Press, 1986).

34. See Leonore Davidoff and Catherine Hall, '"The Hidden Investment": Women and the Enterprise', in Pamela Sharpe (ed.), *Women's Work: The English Experience 1650–1914* (London: Arnold, 1998).

35. See Angus McLaren, *Reproductive Rituals* (London and New York: Methuen, 1984).

36. Granville, Augustus Bozzi, *A Report of the Practice of Midwifery at the Westminster General Dispensary, During 1818; including new classification of labours, abortions, female complaints, etc....*(London: Burgess and Hill, 1819), p. 14. Dispensaries pre-dated hospitals, having been set up in the late seventeenth century to provide advice and medicine to the poor. The first lying-in hospital in England was the British Lying-in Hospital, founded in 1747. A second lying-in hospital was created in the City of London in 1750, and the General Lying-in Hospital was founded in Westminster in 1752. As Wilson has shown, such hospitals had a high profile (and an important role in spreading knowledge and practice), but delivered only a tiny minority (perhaps 5 per cent) of births. See Wilson, *The Making of Man-Midwifery*, p. 146.

37. See John R. Gillis, *For Better, For Worse: British Marriages 1600 to the Present* (New York and Oxford: Oxford University Press, 1985), pp. 126–7 for a discussion of 'proving'.

38. Nicholas Rogers, 'Carnal Knowledge: Illegitimacy in Eighteenth-Century Westminster', *Journal of Social History* 23 (1989), quoted in Robert B. Shoemaker, *Gender in English Society 1650–1850: The Emergence of Separate Spheres?* (Harlow: Longman, 1998), p. 98.

39. See Rogers, in Shoemaker, *Gender in English Society*, p. 99.

40. Angus McLaren, *Reproductive Rituals: The Perception of Fertility in England from the Sixteenth Century to the Nineteenth Century* (London and New York: Methuen, 1984), p. 122.

41. See Barbara Taylor, *Mary Wollstonecraft and the Feminist Imagination* (Cambridge: Cambridge University Press, 2003) for a detailed consideration of Wollstonecraft's religious beliefs.

42. Thomas Laqueur, 'Bodies, Details, and the Humanitarian Narrative', in Lynn Hunt (ed.), *The New Cultural History* (Berkeley and London: University of California Press), 1989.

43. William Hunter, *Anatomia Uteri Humani Gravidi: Tabulis Illustrata* (Birmingham; John Baskerville, 1774), pp. 9–10. Subsequent references are incorporated into the text.

44. Frances Sheridan, *Memoirs of Miss Sidney Bidulph* (1761) (Oxford: Oxford World's Classics, 1999), p. 291.

45. Charlotte Smith, *Montalbert: A Novel*, 3 vols (London: E. Booker, 1795).

46. See Ellen Moers, *Literary Women* (New York: Doubleday, 1977); Mary Jacobus, 'Is There a Woman in This Text?', *New Literary History* 14 (1982), pp. 117–41; Barbara Johnson, *A World of Difference* (Baltimore and London: Johns Hopkins University Press, 1987); and Alan Bewell, 'An Issue of

Monstrous Desire: *Frankenstein* and Obstetrics', *Yale Journal of Criticism* 2, 1 (1988). Moers emphasises Shelley's anxiety in relation to pregnancy. Her first child died within a month of birth, her second child, William, died at the age of three, and her third child lived only a few months. Only one child, her son Percy, survived to adulthood.
47. Mary Shelley, *Frankenstein: or The Modern Prometheus* (1818), ed. Maurice Hindle (Harmondsworth: Penguin, 1992), p. 53. This text is based on the third (1831) edition.
48. See Jacobus, 'Is There a Woman in This Text?'; and Elizabeth Bronfen, *Over Her Dead Body: Death, Femininity and the Aesthetic* (Manchester: Manchester University Press, 1992), p. 131.
49. Mary Wollstonecraft wrote this letter when she was living in Paris during the Reign of the Terror. As with so many aspects of her life and death, her situation here can be all too easily assimilated to myth. It was J.E.D. Esquirol, who worked in the Salpetrière asylum in Paris and took a particular interest in insanity in pregnancy, who made the influential suggestion that the children of those mothers who were pregnant in the revolutionary period were particularly vulnerable to insanity in later life. He attributed this to the stress they were under *in utero*, which was communicated to them by their mother. It became commonplace to refer to this idea in nineteenth-century textbooks of obstetrics; see, for example, George Man Burrows, *Commentaries on the Causes, Forms, Symptoms, and Treatment, Moral and Medical, of Insanity* (London: Thomas and George Underwood, 1828). The child for whom Mary was anxious, Fanny Imlay, suffered from periods of depression and committed suicide in 1816 when she discovered that she was illegitimate. Her 'insanity' was probably largely due to the cruelty and indifference of her stepmother: none the less, it has a poignant resonance in the light of contemporary myths (and fears) about pregnancy.

Chapter 2

1. Robert Owen, *Lectures on the Marriages of the Priesthood of the Old Immoral World* (1840), quoted in Kathryn Gleadle (ed.), *Radical Writing on Women, 1800–1850: An Anthology* (Basingstoke: Palgrave Macmillan, 2002), p.135.
2. Richard Carlile, *Every Woman's Book; or, What is Love?* (London: published by the author, 1828), pp. 25–6. Subsequent references are incorporated into the text.
3. Barbara Taylor, *Eve and the New Jerusalem* (London: Virago, 1983), pp. 47–8.
4. Robert Dale Owen, *Moral Physiology; or, a Brief and Plain Treatise on The Population Question* (1830) (London: J. Watson, 1846), p. 1. Subsequent references are incorporated into the text. Although Dale Owen emigrated to America, he maintained strong links with friends and colleagues in Britain, and his work was influential in the UK.
5. Emma Martin, *The Bible No Revelation, or the Inadequacy of Language to Convey a Message from God to Man*, second edition (London: published by the author, c.1850), n.p.
6. As the debate over female sexual passivity demonstrates, no view escaped discussion and contestation in the medical community, particularly as the

influence of journals such as the *Edinburgh Medical Journal* and the *Lancet* grew.

7. John Power, *Essays on the Female Economy* (London: Burgess and Hill, 1821), p. 11. Subsequent references are incorporated into the text.

8. O. Moscucci, *The Science of Woman: Gynaecology and Gender in England, 1800–1929* (Cambridge: Cambridge University Press, 1990), p. 25.

9. Alexander Walker, *Woman, Physiologically Considered as to Mind, Morals, Marriage, Matrimonial Slavery, Infidelity and Divorce* (1839) (London: A.H. Baily & Co., 1840), pp. 23–4. Subsequent references are incorporated into the text.

10. See Jill L. Matus, *Unstable Bodies: Victorian Representations of Sexuality and Maternity* (Manchester: Manchester University Press, 1995), p. 31.

11. William Acton, *The Functions and Disorders of the Reproductive Organs in Childhood, Youth, Adult Age, and Advanced Life, Considered in their Physiological, Social, and Moral Relations* (1857) (London: J. and A. Churchill, 1875), pp. 212 and 183. Subsequent references are incorporated into the text.

12. Thomas Laycock, *Mind and Brain: or, The Correlations of Consciousness and Organisation: Systematically Investigated and Applied to Philosophy, Mental Science and Practice* (London: Simpkin, Marshall and Co., 1869), quoted in Ellen Wood, *East Lynne* (1861), ed. Andrew Maunder (Peterborough, Ontario: Broadview Literary Texts, 2000), p. 734.

13. W. Tyler Smith, *A Manual of Obstetrics: Theoretical and Practical* (London: John Churchill, 1858), p. 28.

14. See, for example, Elaine Showalter, *The Female Malady: Women, Madness and English Culture, 1830–1980* (London: Virago, 1987).

15. See, for example, Joan Jacobs Brumberg, *Fasting Girls: The Emergence of Anorexia Nervosa as a Modern Disease* (Cambridge, Mass. and London: Harvard University Press, 1988).

16. Nancy Theriot, 'Diagnosing Unnatural Motherhood: Nineteenth-century Physicians and "Puerperal Insanity"', in Philip K. Wilson (ed.), *Childbirth: Changing Ideas and Practices in Britain and America 1600 to the Present* (New York and London: Garland Publishing, 1996), Vol. 5, pp. 133–52.

17. Douglas Fox, *The Signs, Disorders and Management of Pregnancy: the Treatment to be Adopted During and After Confinement; and the Management and Disorders of Children .Written Expressly for the Use of Females* (Derby: Henry Mozley & Sons, 1834), p. 2. Subsequent references will be incorporated into the text.

18. W.F. Montgomery, *An Exposition of the Signs and Symptoms of Pregnancy, the Period of Human Gestation, and the Signs of Delivery* (London: Sherwood, Gilbert, & Piper, 1837), pp. 18–20.

19. James Cowles Pritchard, *A Treatise on Insanity and Other Disorders Affecting the Mind* (London: Sherwood, Gilbert, and Piper, 1835), p. 306.

20. George Man Burrows, *Commentaries on the Causes, Forms, Symptoms, and Treatment, Moral and Medical, of Insanity* (London: Thomas and George Underwood, 1828), pp. 363–4.

21. Robert Lee, *Three Hundred Consultations in Midwifery* (London: John Churchill and Sons, 1864), pp. 21–2.

22. J.B. Tuke, 'On the Statistics of Puerperal Insanity as observed in the Royal Edinburgh Asylum, Morningside', *Edinburgh Medical Journal*, Vol. X (July

1864–June 1865; Edinburgh: Oliver and Boyd, 1865), pp. 1015–16. Subsequent references are incorporated into the text.

23. Henry Maudsley, *The Physiology and Pathology of Mind*, second edition (London: Macmillan and Co., 1868), p. 399.

24. W.S. Playfair, *A Treatise on the Science and Practice of Midwifery*, third edition (London: Smith, Elder, & Co., 1880), pp. 312–13.

25. Thomas John Graham, *Modern Domestic Medicine*, second edition (London: Simpkin & Marshall, 1827), pp. 397–9. As Sally Shuttleworth has pointed out, Graham's book constituted a 'secular Bible' for the Brontës' father, the Reverend Patrick Brontë. He took a keen interest in medical matters, and almost every page of his copy is covered with annotations querying interpretations and recording alternative remedies. See Sally Shuttleworth, *Charlotte Brontë and Victorian Psychology* (Cambridge: Cambridge University Press, 1996), p. 27.

26. Sandra M. Gilbert and Susan Gubar, *The Madwoman in the Attic: The Woman Writer and the Nineteenth-Century Literary Imagination*, second edition (New Haven and London: Yale University Press, 2000), p. 272.

27. Emily Brontë, *Wuthering Heights* (1847) (Harmondsworth: Penguin, 1988), p. 93. Subsequent references are incorporated into the text.

28. Eugenie Lemione-Luccioni, *The Dividing of Women or Woman's Lot* (*Partage des Femmes*), trans. Marie-Laure Davenport and Marie-Christine Reguis (London: Free Association Books, 1987), p. 33. Subsequent references are incorporated into the text.

29. See Elaine Showalter, *The Female Malady: Women, Madness and English Culture, 1830–1980* (London: Virago, 1987), p.10 for a discussion of this.

30. Angela Carter, *Nights at the Circus* (London: Vintage, [1984] 1994), p. 190.

31. In nineteenth-century psychiatry it was often argued that mental disorders had their origins in organic disease, and brain inflammation, or fever, was often cited as a cause of such disorders. See Roy Porter, *The Greatest Benefit to Mankind: A Medical History of Humanity from Antiquity to the Present* (London: Fontana Press, 1999), pp. 508–9.

32. Introduction to Ellen Wood, *East Lynne*, ed. Andrew Maunder, pp. 17 and 9.

33. Ibid., p. 374. Subsequent references are incorporated into the text.

34. It had previously been thought that female sexual pleasure, or 'heat', was necessary for conception, and this belief lingered in the popular imagination. As W.F. Montgomery notes, in the past this had serious implications in cases of rape which resulted in pregnancy, for this was 'presumed to prove consent' (*Signs and Symptoms*, p. 199).

35. Elizabeth Barrett-Browning, *Aurora Leigh* (1857), ed. Cora Kaplan (London: The Women's Press, 1978), p. 280.

36. See Barbara Taylor, *Eve and the New Jerusalem* (London: Virago, 1983), p. 201.

37. For details of the case, see J.A.V. Chapple and Arthur Pollard (eds), *The Letters of Mrs Gaskell* (Manchester: Manchester University Press, 1966), pp. 98–100.

38. W.R. Greg, 'The False Morality of Lady Novelists', published in *The National Review* in January 1859, quoted in the Introduction to Elizabeth Gaskell, *Ruth*, ed. Alan Shelston (Oxford: World's Classics, 1998), p. xiv. Greg was a Unitarian intellectual known personally to Gaskell. He was best known for

his influential article on prostitution, published in the *Westminster Review* in 1850. In this he expressed the somewhat patronising view that the majority of prostitutes and kept women 'fall in the first instance from a mere exaggeration and perversion of one of the best qualities of a woman's heart. They yield to desires in which they do not share, from a weak generosity which cannot refuse anything to the passionate entreaties of the man they love' (quoted in Janet Horowitz Murray (ed.), *Strong-Minded Women* (Harmondsworth: Penguin, 1984), p. 410).

39. See, for example, Caroline Norton's poem on the seduction theme, 'The Sorrows of Rosalie', reprinted in Isobel Armstrong, Joseph Bristow and Cath Sharrock (eds), *Nineteenth-Century Women Poets: An Oxford Anthology* (Oxford: Clarendon Press, 1996), pp. 327–9.

40. Gaskell, *Ruth*, p. 45. Subsequent references are incorporated into the text. Gaskell's novel may also have been influenced in part by Nathaniel Hawthorne's *The Scarlet Letter* (1850), which she is likely to have read.

41. See Deborah Cherry, *Painting Women: Victorian Women Artists* (London: Routledge, 1993), pp. 154–7. Cherry discusses visual images of the seamstress produced by men and women painters. Thomas Hood's poem 'The Song of the Shirt', on the sufferings of needlewomen, was first published in *Punch* in 1843.

42. Sarah Lewis, *Woman's Mission* (London: J.W. Parker, 1839), p. 21.

43. Josephine Butler, 'The Education and Employment of Women', first published in 1868, reprinted in *Strong-Minded Women*, p. 219.

44. George Eliot, *Adam Bede* (1859) (New York: Random House, 2002), p. 152. Subsequent references are incorporated into the text. It is worth noting that Walter Scott's *Heart of Midlothian* is an important pre-text for *Adam Bede* in its treatment of the theme of infanticide.

45. Eliot was familiar with versions of evolutionary thought which antedated the publication of *The Origin of Species*. When she first met her partner, George Henry Lewes, he was writing on 'the Development Hypothesis' with reference to Lyell and Owen. Herbert Spencer also published on the 'Development Hypothesis', and applied evolutionary theory to the human mind in his *Principles of Psychology* (1855).

46. Eliot was criticised in some quarters for giving too much detail about Hetty's experience of pregnancy. The *Saturday Review* thought that the descriptions of her pregnancy 'read like the rough notes of a man-midwife's conversation with a bride' and asked for a return to earlier traditions: 'Let us copy the old masters of the art, who, if they gave us a baby, gave it us all at once.' One of the strengths of the novel, however, is Eliot's representation of pregnancy as an experience of duration and process. James Simpson, the Professor of Midwifery at Edinburgh, strongly endorsed the novel's sympathetic power when it was sent to him by Eliot's publisher, who was seeking reassurance that the novel did not offend against decency. Simpson pointed out, however, that a child as premature as Hetty's would have been too weak to cry as it does in the novel. See Gordon Haight, *George Eliot: A Biography* (Oxford: Clarendon Press, 1968); and David Carroll (ed.), *George Eliot: The Critical Heritage* (London: Routledge and Kegan Paul, 1971).

47. Leigh Summers, *Bound to Please: A History of the Victorian Corset* (Oxford: Berg, 2001), p. 50. Summers suggests that corsets may have been deliber-

ately adopted not only to disguise pregnancy but to terminate it, through the pressure they exerted on the foetus. Discussing this issue in 1904, however, J.W. Ballantyne concluded that 'the writers who have so emphatically condemned the corset as "the evil of the age," and the active cause of pelvic congestion, of defective secretion of bile, of dyspepsia and the like, have little or nothing to say of its teratogenic influence upon the unborn infant. One is driven to the conclusion that its ill-effects, in this direction at least, are few; perhaps the presence of the liquor amnii is the great safeguard of the foetus.' *Manual of Antenatal Pathology and Hygiene: The Embryo* (Edinburgh: William Green & Sons, 1904), pp. 139–40.

48. Henry Pye Chavasse, *Advice to a Wife on the Management of her Own Health and on the Treatment of Some of the Complaints Incidental to Pregnancy, Labour, and Suckling, with an Introductory Chapter Especially Addressed to a Young Wife*, twelfth edition (London: J. and A. Churchill, 1877), p. 125. This advice book was hugely popular and went through sixteen editions between its first publication in 1847 and 1914.

49. William Hunter, 'On the Uncertainty of the Signs of Murder in the Case of Bastard Children' (London: J. Callow, 1812), pp. 9–10.

50. There was great concern about this issue in the 1850s. Eliot based her novel in part on a story told to her by her aunt, about the trial of a young woman for child-murder earlier in the century. However, she would also have been aware of cases such as that of Maria Clarke, who was convicted of murdering her illegitimate child in 1851: like Hetty, she had buried her child alive. Her sentence was later commuted by the Home Secretary. Books began to appear on the subject in the 1860s, including William B. Ryan's *Infanticide: Its Law, Prevalence, Prevention and History* (London: Churchill, 1862). See Matus, *Unstable Bodies* for a helpful discussion of this issue.

51. See Judith Schneid Lewis, *In the Family Way: Childbearing in the British Aristocracy, 1760–1860* (New Brunswick: Rutgers University Press, 1986), p. 124.

52. Quoted in Joan Perkin, *Victorian Women* (London: John Murray, 1993), p. 66.

53. Roger Fulford (ed.), *Dearest Child: Letters between Queen Victoria and the Princess Royal, 1858–1861* (London: Evans Brothers, 1964), pp. 77–8, letter of 15 March 1858.

54. Ibid., p. 115, letter of 15 June 1858.

55. Ibid., p. 195, letter of 15 June 1859.

56. See Mary Russo, *The Female Grotesque: Risk, Excess and Modernity* (London: Routledge, 1994), p. 8.

Chapter 3

1. These statistics are taken from Ann Oakley, *The Captured Womb: A History of the Medical Care of Pregnant Women* (Oxford: Blackwell, 1984), pp. 37 and 296.

2. From an article by J.L. Garvin, quoted in Anna Davin, 'Imperialism and Motherhood', *History Workshop* Vol. 5 (Spring 1978), p. 10.

3. See Oakley, *The Captured Womb*, pp. 35–6, for a discussion of this.
4. For example, in his *Principles of Mental Physiology*, William Carpenter writes of the 'Race' in terms that suggest that he means by this all the Anglo-Saxon races. See *The Principles of Mental Physiology*, third edition (London: J. and A. Churchill, 1875), p. 368. By contrast, Elizabeth Blackwell (an American living in Britain) ties the concept of 'the race' closely to the individual nation state in *The Human Element in Sex: Being a Medical Enquiry into the Relation of Sexual Physiology to Christian Morality* (London: J. and A. Churchill, 1894), p. 28.
5. Extract from Francis Galton, *Inquiries into Human Faculty and Its Development*, in Laura Otis (ed.), *Literature and Science in the Nineteenth Century* (Oxford: Oxford World's Classics, 2002), p. 479.
6. See Max Nordau, *Degeneration*, trans. from the second edition of the German (London: William Heinemann, 1895), pp. 16 and 34. Nordau argues that degenerates will be unable to adapt and maintain themselves in the struggle for existence: 'That which distinguishes degeneracy from the formation of new species (phylogeny) is, that the morbid variation does not continuously subsist and propagate itself, like one that is healthy, but, for-tunately, is soon rendered sterile, and after a few generations often dies out before it reaches the lowest grade of organic degradation' (p. 16).
7. J.W. Ballantyne, *Expectant Motherhood: Its Supervision and Hygiene* (London, New York, Toronto and Melbourne: Cassell & Co., 1914), p. 98. Subsequent references are incorporated into the text.
8. Pauline Mazumdar, *Eugenics, Human Genetics and Human Failings* (London: Routledge, 1992), p. 85.
9. Quoted in Janet Horowitz Murray (ed.), *Strong-Minded Women* (Harmondsworth: Penguin, 1984), p. 221.
10. Quoted ibid., p. 223.
11. S. Weir Mitchell, *Wear and Tear, or Hints for the Overworked*, fifth edition (Philadelphia: J.B. Lippincott Company, 1887), pp. 43–4. It is worth noting that this was a period of rapidly increasing communication and exchange of ideas between British and American physicians. Specialist journals were subscribed to on both sides of the Atlantic, and medical textbooks were often published in both countries.
12. Caleb Williams Saleeby, *Woman and Womanhood: A Search for Principles* (London: William Heinemann, 1912), p. 7.
13. Marie Stopes, *Wise Parenthood* (1918), twelfth edition (London: G.P. Putnam's Sons, 1926), pp. 1–2.
14. Quoted in Robert A. Peel (ed.), *Essays in the History of Eugenics* (London: The Galton Institute, 1998), p. 39.
15. It was Grand who, with Ouida, coined the term 'New Woman' to denote the intelligent, independent woman of the period, whose desires and demands were closely linked with the women's suffrage movement.
16. Sarah Grand, *The Heavenly Twins* (1893) (London: William Heinemann, 1895), p. 185. Subsequent references are incorporated into the text.
17. Grand's novel was published two years before Freud and Breuer's first case histories appeared in *Studien über Hysterie* (1895).
18. Henry Maudsley, *The Pathology of Mind*, quoted in Elaine Showalter, *The Female Malady: Women, Madness and English Culture, 1830–1980* (London: Virago, 1987, p. 130.

19. W.F. Dakin, *A Handbook of Midwifery* (London, New York and Bombay: Longmans, Green and Co., 1897), pp. 556–7.
20. George Egerton, *Keynotes and Discords* (1893) (London: Virago, 1983), p. 2. Subsequent references are incorporated into the text.
21. Charles Darwin, *The Descent of Man and Selection in Relation to Sex* (1871) (New York: Hurst and Company, 1875), p. 618. Subsequent references are incorporated into the text.
22. J.W. Ballantyne, 'A Plea for a Pro-Maternity Hospital', *British Medical Journal* (6 April 1901), p. 813.
23. As Ann Oakley explains, Ballantyne used the prefix 'pro' in the Greek sense meaning 'before', not the Latin 'in favour of'. However, his terminology caused confusion, and he reverted to the prefix 'pre' in later writings. As Oakley also notes, Ballantyne was something of a polymath, part of 'the international academic community', and able to lecture in Latin to international students. He also had an interest in medical history, and published a study of the various extant editions of Reynalde's *The Byrth of Mankynde*, the first midwifery text in English. See the pamphlet reprinted from the *Journal of Obstetrics and Gynaecology of the British Empire*, 'The "Byrth of Mankynde" (Its Author and Editions)' (London and Manchester: Sherratt and Hughes, 1906).
24. The understanding of the relationship between mother and foetus in terms of competition rather than symbiosis will be discussed in chapter 5. See also David Barker, *The Best Start in Life: How a Woman's Diet Can Protect her Child from Disease in Later Life* (London: Century Books, 2003), pp. 92–4.
25. Evelyn M. Bunting (ed.), *A School for Mothers* (London: Horace Marshall and Son, 1907), p. 5. Subsequent references will be incorporated into the text.
26. In her polemical work *Save the Mothers* (discussed in the next chapter), Sylvia Pankhurst deploys a still more emotive image of the starving pregnant woman driven to theft: 'Back through the years there flashes on me the vision of a cold grey morning in smoke-ridden Manchester: I in the Oxford Road on my way to school, a woman in a shawl, gauntly emaciated, yet big with child. She stretches a fleshless arm to take from the butcher's board a long bone, utterly meatless. Two well-groomed gentlemen, one with a tall hat, pass me and break into a run, seizing her a few paces from the shop. She turns to them a haggard and tragic face. The butcher runs out, a crowd gathers, a policeman appears.' *Save the Mothers* (London: Alfred A. Knopf, 1930), p. 26.
27. For a thoughtful discussion of class-bias at the School for Mothers, see Anna Davin, 'Imperialism and Motherhood'. As she points out, although workers for the School were class-bound in many respects, they succeeded, in large part, because they did assume goodwill in the mothers.
28. Anna Wickham, 'Fragment of an Autobiography', reprinted in R.D. Smith (ed.), *The Writings of Anna Wickham, Free Woman and Poet* (London: Virago, 1984), p. 148.
29. Anna Wickham, 'Lecture: School for Mothers', reprinted in Smith, *The Writings of Anna Wickham*, p. 372 (date of delivery not known). Subsequent references will be incorporated into the text.
30. Preface to Margaret Llewelyn Davies (ed.), *Maternity: Letters from Working Women* (1915) (London: Virago, 1978). Subsequent references will be incorporated into the text.

31. Abortifacients fell into two broad categories in this period. Those available over the chemist's counter, such as Epsom salts or castor oil, were usually both harmless and ineffective. Far more dangerous were those remedies based on lead which could bring about insanity or death. These circulated under such euphemistic names as 'Mrs Seagrave's pills' and 'Nurse O's pills'.
32. Oakley, *The Captured Womb*, p. 54.
33. Charlotte Perkins Gilman, *Herland* (1915) (London: The Women's Press, 1979), pp. 68–70. Subsequent references will be incorporated into the text.
34. For a discussion of Barrett's views, see Lesley A. Hall, 'Women, Feminism and Eugenics', in Robert A. Peel (ed.), *Essays in the History of Eugenics* (London: The Galton Institute, 1998).
35. See August Weismann, *Essays upon Heredity and Kindred Biological Problems*, 2 vols (Oxford: Clarendon Press, 1889–92). Weismann contended that an immutable 'germ plasm' passed from generation to generation, unmodified by experience or environment.
36. Sigmund Freud and Joseph Breuer, *Studies on Hysteria*, Penguin Freud Library 3 (Harmondsworth: Penguin, 1988), p. 95.
37. Quoted in Mikkel Borch-Jacobsen, *Remembering Anna O: A Century of Mystification*, trans. Kirby Olson in collaboration with Xavier Callahan and the author (New York and London: Routledge, 1996), p. 29.
38. Quoted ibid., p. 100.
39. Ernest Jones, *The Young Freud, 1856–1900* (London: Hogarth Press, 1956), p. 247, emphasis added.
40. Quoted in Lisa Appignanesi and John Forrester, *Freud's Women* (London: Virago, 1993), p. 81.
41. See *Remembering Anna O: A Century of Mystification* and *Freud's Women*, for detailed discussions of source and archive material in relation to this case.
42. See Michel Foucault, *The History of Sexuality: Volume One, An Introduction* (1976) (Harmondsworth: Penguin, 1990), for his account of 'the repressive hypothesis', in which he argues that speaking of what is culturally forbidden itself generates 'effects of power' (p. 11).
43. Juliet Mitchell, *Mad Men and Medusas: Reclaiming Hysteria and the Effects of Sibling Relations on the Human Condition* (Harmondsworth: Penguin, 2000), p. 155.
44. See Helene Deutsch, 'The Psychology of Women in Relation to the Functions of Reproduction' (1924), in R. Fliess, *The Psychoanalytic Reader* (London: Hogarth Press, 1950); Karen Horney, 'The Flight from Womanhood' (1926), in *Feminine Psychology* (New York: Norton, 1967).
45. For an early account of Lawrence's knowledge of Freud and Freudianism, see Emile Delavenay, *D. H. Lawrence: The Man and His Work, The Formative Years: 1885–1919* (London: Heinemann, 1972). See also George J. Zytaruk and James T. Boulton (eds), *The Letters of D.H. Lawrence, Vol. 11, 1913–15* (Cambridge: Cambridge University Press, 1981).
46. D.H. Lawrence, *The Rainbow* (1915) (Harmondsworth: Penguin, 1972), p. 64. Subsequent references are incorporated into the text.
47. The essay is reprinted in *The Writings of Anna Wickham*, pp. 355–72. Wickham may have been one of the models for the character of Anna Brangwen (alternatively, Wickham may have re-cast her maternal experiences in the light of her reading of Lawrence). In her memoir, she writes of

her third (and first successful) pregnancy in these terms: 'I experienced a sort of glorification at my condition; "Blessed art thou among Women". I took my harmony exercises to the beach and worked as far as 'suspensions' as preparation for the songs I would write, but the child in my womb came between me and my music ... The day of this son's birth was the happiest of my life. This was the self-expression which I believed in, and which gave me delight. As I lay after my labour, clean, completed, with the child on my arm, I felt something that was like physical passion for the first time since my marriage' (pp. 146–7). She adds: 'The only aspect of physical love that interested me was impregnation, and constantly and conscientiously I became impregnated. I then had no doubt whatever of my right to it' (p. 150).

48. Quoted in Maud Ellmann, *The Hunger Artists: Starving, Writing and Imprisonment* (London: Virago, 1993), p. 44.
49. Katherine Mansfield, *In a German Pension* (1911) (Harmondsworth: Penguin, 1975), pp. 38–9.
50. Katherine Mansfield, *Selected Stories* (Oxford: Oxford World's Classics, 1981), p. 77. Subsequent references will be incorporated into the text.

Chapter 4

1. J.B.S. Haldane, *Daedalus or Science and the Future* (London: Kegan Paul, Trench, Trubner & Co. Ltd., 1924); Ronald C. Macfie, *Metanthropos, or the Future of the Body* (London: Kegan Paul, Trench, Trubner & Co. Ltd., 1928); Garet Garrett, *Ouroboros, of the Mechanical Extension of Mankind* (London: Kegan Paul, Trench, Trubner & Co. Ltd, 1926). These were all published in the 'Today and Tomorrow' series.
2. I am using problematic in the sense in which it is used by Mazumdar, to denote 'a field of concepts which organises a particular science by making it possible to ask some kinds of questions and suppressing others'. See Pauline Mazumdar, *Eugenics, Human Genetics and Human Failings* (London: Routledge, 1992), p. 1.
3. Grantly Dick Read, *Revelation of Childbirth* (London: Heinemann, 1942), published in the US in 1944 as *Childbirth Without Fear* (this was the title which was subsequently adopted in Britain).
4. See Patricia Romero, *E. Sylvia Pankhurst: Portrait of a Radical* (New Haven and London: Yale University Press, 1987), p. 168.
5. *News of the World* (8 April 1928), p. 1.
6. Sylvia Pankhurst, *Save the Mothers* (London: Knopf, 1930), p. 33.
7. See Pauline Mazumdar, *Eugenics, Human Genetics and Human Failings* (London: Routledge, 1992), p. 178.
8. Ibid., p. 210.
9. Enid Bagnold, *The Squire* (1938) (London: Virago, 1987), p. 88. Subsequent references will be incorporated into the text.
10. The letter from Wells is quoted in Anne Sebba, *Enid Bagnold: The Authorized Biography* (London: Weidenfeld and Nicolson, 1986), p. 137.
11. See, for example, Janet Campbell, who in *The Protection of Motherhood* (London: HMSO, 1927) implicitly aligns mothers and soldiers when she

argues that 'much can be done ... to direct attention to the importance of saving and safeguarding the Nation's mothers and of giving them sympathetic and effective support in their arduous and sometimes perilous task of maintaining the race' (p. 71).

12. Quoted in Sebba, *Enid Bagnold*, p. 141. See ibid., pp. 138–43 for a discussion of Bagnold's response to Hitler's Germany. In relation to this, see also Clare Hanson, 'Save the Mothers? Representations of Pregnancy in the 1930s', *Literature and History* 12, 2 (Autumn 2003).

13. G.F. McCleary, *Race Suicide?* (London: George Allen and Unwin Ltd, 1945), pp. 87–9.

14. Grace Leybourne-White and Kenneth White, *Children for Britain* (London: Pilot Press, 1945), p. 16. Subsequent references are incorporated into the text.

15. Royal Commission on Population, *Report* (London: HMSO, 1949), p. 134.

16. It should be noted that both J.B.S. Haldane and his sister Naomi (the novelist Naomi Mitchison) were members of the Eugenics Society before the First World War: both subsequently became extremely critical of class-based eugenics.

17. See Mazumdar, *Eugenics, Human Genetics and Human Failings*, p. 182, for further discussion of Haldane's work on evolutionary change.

18. Among the best known of these books are *Daedalus* (1924), *Possible Worlds* (1927), *Heredity and Politics* (1938) and *Science and Everyday Life* (1939).

19. J.B.S. Haldane, *Daedalus or Science and the Future* (London: Kegan Paul, Trench, Trubner & Co., Ltd, 1924), p. 64. Subsequent references are incorporated into the text.

20. See Charlotte Haldane, *Truth Will Out* (London: Weidenfeld and Nicolson, 1949) for an account of her meeting with and marriage to Haldane.

21. Charlotte Haldane, *Man's World* (London: Chatto and Windus, 1926), p. 9. Subsequent references are incorporated into the text.

22. Charlotte Haldane, *Motherhood and Its Enemies* (London: Chatto and Windus, 1927), p. 238. Subsequent references are incorporated into the text.

23. See Jane Lewis, *The Politics of Motherhood* (London: Croom Helm, 1980); and Susan Merrill Squier, *Babies in Bottles: Twentieth-Century Visions of Reproductive Technology* (New Brunswick: Rutgers University Press, 1994).

24. Aldous Huxley, 'A Note on Eugenics', in *Proper Studies* (London: Chatto and Windus, 1927).

25. Aldous Huxley, *Brave New World* (1932), with an introduction by David Bradshaw (London: Flamingo, 1994), p. 8. Subsequent references will be incorporated into the text.

26. The Haldanes first visited Russia in the 1930s and were enthusiastic about the 'social experiment' taking place there; Aldous Huxley expressed his support for 'something on the lines of ' the Russian Five-Year Plan in a letter to his father of August 1931 (quoted in Bradshaw's introduction to *Brave New World*).

27. *The Queen Charlotte's Practice of Obstetrics* (London: J. and A. Churchill, 1927), p. 73.

28. Eardley Holland, R.C. Jewsbury and Wilfred Sheldon, *A Doctor to a Mother: The Management of Maternal and Infant Health* (London: Edward Arnold,

1933), p. 8, emphasis added. Holland wrote the section on pregnancy for this small paperback, which was based on radio talks.

29. Ann Oakley, *The Captured Womb: A History of the Medical Care of Pregnant Women* (Oxford: Blackwell, 1984), p. 252.
30. F.J. Browne, *Antenatal and Postnatal Care* (London: J. and A. Churchill, 1935), pp. 17–18, emphasis added.
31. Quoted in Janelle S. Taylor, 'Of Sonograms and Baby Prams: Prenatal Diagnosis, Pregnancy, and Consumption', *Feminist Studies* 26, 2 (Summer 2000), p. 395.
32. Margery Spring Rice, *Working-Class Wives: Their Health and Conditions*, with an introduction by Dame Janet Campbell (Harmondsworth: Penguin, 1939), p. 47. Subsequent references are incorporated into the text.
33. Oakley, *The Captured Womb*, p. 125.
34. Quoted in ibid., pp. 124–5. As Oakley points out, it was not just the 'income- and diet-equalizing policies' of the wartime government which were responsible for the improved health of mothers and children. The underlying trend towards more national health care, and longer-term changes in the ages and obstetric health of mothers, were also important factors.
35. The National Health Service Act was passed in 1946 in England and 1947 in Scotland. It came into operation on 5 July 1948.
36. Joint Committee of the Royal College of Obstetricians and Gynaecologists and the Population Investigation Committee, *Maternity in Great Britain* (Oxford: Oxford University Press, 1948), p. 45. Subsequent references are incorporated into the text.
37. Sarah Campion, *National Baby* (London: Ernest Benn, 1950), p. 141. Subsequent references are incorporated into the text.
38. A.S. Byatt, *Still Life* (1985) (Harmondsworth: Penguin, 1986), p. 16. Subsequent references are incorporated into the text.
39. Quoted in W.F. Bynum and Roy Porter (eds), *William Hunter and the Eighteenth-Century Medical World* (Cambridge: Cambridge University Press, 1985), p. 362.
40. Norman Morris, 'Human Relations in Obstetric Practice', *The Lancet*, Vol. 1 (January–June 1960), p. 913. See also Michel Foucault, *The Birth of the Clinic: An Archaeology of Medical Perception*, trans. A.M. Sheridan (London: Routledge, 1997), p. 14.
41. See Christopher Lawrence, *Medicine in the Making of Modern Britain 1700–1920* (London: Routledge, 1994), pp. 86–7.
42. Dugald Baird, 'The Evolution of Modern Obstetrics', *The Lancet*, Vol. 2 (July–December 1960), p. 560.
43. Ibid., pp. 612–13.
44. Marion H. Hall, P.K. Ching and I. MacGillivray, 'Is Routine Antenatal Care Worthwhile?', *The Lancet*, Vol. 2 (July–December 1980), pp. 78–80. The authors concluded that it was not: 'The productivity of routine antenatal care in respect of prediction and detection of obstetric problems is extremely low, and it is suggested that the number of visits for this purpose could be considerably reduced for women without special problems' (p. 78).
45. A.S. Byatt, *The Virgin in the Garden* (1978) (Harmondsworth: Penguin, 1981), p. 295.
46. These figures are taken from Oakley, *The Captured Womb*, p. 105.

47. Stuart Campbell (ed.), *Ultrasound in Obstetrics and Gynaecology: Recent Advances*, book version of *Clinics in Obstetrics and Gynaecology*, Vol. 10, No. 3 (December 1983) (London, Philadelphia and Toronto: W.B. Saunders, 1983), p. 369. Subsequent references are incorporated into the text.

48. Joanna Moorhead, *New Generations: 40 Years of Birth in Britain* (Cambridge: HMSO in collaboration with National Childbirth Trust Publishing Ltd., 1996), p. 25.

49. Grantly Dick Read, *Natural Childbirth* (London: William Heinemann, 1933), p. 37.

50. Read, *Revelation of Childbirth*, pp. 73–4.

51. Ibid., p. 88.

52. Read, *Natural Childbirth*, p. 23.

53. Ibid., p. 44.

54. American obstetricians were far less sympathetic to Read's ideas. The most damaging attack on his work came in a 1950 article in the *Journal of the American Medical Association* which challenged Read's claim that women of more 'primitive' societies had less painful labours. The authors disputed the idea that pain was caused by fear, and that education about childbirth eliminated pain: they also argued that interventionist modern obstetrics had brought about a reduction in maternal and infant mortality. See D. Reid and M.E. Cohen, 'Trends in Obstetrics', *Journal of the American Medical Association*, Vol. 142 (1950), pp. 615–23.

55. See Julia Kristeva, 'Motherhood According to Giovanni Bellini' (1975); 'Stabat Mater' (1977); and 'Women's Time' (1979), all in Kelly Oliver (ed.), *The Portable Kristeva* (New York and Chichester: Columbia University Press, 1997).

56. It was the embryologist Ernst Haeckel who first proposed that 'ontogeny [the development of the individual] is a recapitulation of phylogeny [the development of the race]', in *The Evolution of Man* (1874). Freud developed this idea in *Moses and Monotheism* (1932).

57. Doris Lessing, *A Proper Marriage* (1964) (St Albans: Panther Books, 1966), p. 129.

58. Doris Lessing, *Under My Skin: Volume One of My Autobiography, To 1949* (1994) (London: Flamingo, 1995), p. 214.

59. Margaret Hebblethwaite gives this account: 'Antenatal classes with Sheila Kitzinger were something special. She taught in her lovely Cotswold home, in a huge sitting room with lots of arty sofas and bean bags and floor cushions, which created an air of luxury and made you feel pampered. Sheila herself bubbled with enthusiasm and energy, and obviously loved her subject: you couldn't help but be infected with her spirit. At our last class we were pretending to have contractions when one woman began to go into early labour for real. Another woman, whose EDD [estimated delivery date] was supposed to be sooner, sat on the floor next to her and said, "I'm so jealous". We all felt like that. We were looking forward to the great adventure.' Quoted in Moorhead, *New Generations*, p. 62.

60. Marjorie Tew, *Safer Childbirth? A Critical History of Maternity Care*, second edition (London: Chapman and Hall, 1995), p. 235.

61. Sheila Kitzinger, *The Experience of Childbirth*, revised edition (Harmondsworth: Penguin, 1967), p. 19. Subsequent references will be incorporated into the text.

62. It is instructive to compare Kitzinger's discussion of depression in pregnancy with the rather brutalist treatment of the subject in the 1952 edition

of *The Queen Charlotte's Practice of Obstetrics*. In the latter, in a chapter entitled 'Psychiatry and Reproduction', it is claimed that of the psychoses of
pregnancy, depression is by far the most common. If the child is unwanted
(as, for example, in the case of an unmarried mother), this may cause reac-
tive depression. It is noted that manic-depression can also manifest itself in
pregnancy, and should be treated with electro-convulsive therapy, which
can be administered up to the seventh month. In a startlingly crude
reflection of the social prejudices of the day, the medical practitioner is
reminded that 'the unmarried mother will often show some degree of
mental defect or backwardness'. The local Department of Health which
deals with mental deficiency should thus be notified of such cases, so that
these women can receive 'care and supervision' (p. 488).
63. Barbara Creed, 'Horror and the Monstrous-Feminine: An Imaginary
    Abjection', *Screen*, Vol. 27, No. 1 (January–February 1986), pp. 55 and 58.
64. John Wyndham, *The Midwich Cuckoos* (1957) (Harmondsworth: Penguin,
    1960), p. 174. Subsequent references are incorporated into the text.

Chapter 5

1. Shulamith Firestone, *The Dialectic of Sex: The Case for a Feminist Revolution*
   (1970) (London: Jonathan Cape, 1971), p. 8. Subsequent references are
   incorporated into the text.
2. See Germaine Greer, *The Whole Woman* (1999) (London: Anchor, 2000),
   pp. 94–106; E. Ann Kaplan, *Motherhood and Representation: The Mother in
   Popular Culture and Melodrama* (London: Routledge, 1992), pp. 209–15.
3. Susan Himmelweit, 'Abortion: Individual Choice and Social Control'
   (1980), reprinted in Feminist Review Collective (ed.), *Sexuality: A Reader*
   (London: Virago, 1987), p. 99.
4. Quoted in Germaine Greer, *The Female Eunuch* (1970) (London: Flamingo,
   1999), p. 336.
5. Janet Radcliffe Richards, *The Sceptical Feminist: A Philosophical Enquiry* (1980)
   (Harmondsworth: Penguin, 1988), p. 294.
6. Adrienne Rich, *Of Woman Born: Motherhood as Experience and Institution* (1976)
   (London: Virago, 1986), p. 13. Subsequent references will be incorporated
   into the text.
7. Julia Kristeva, 'Motherhood According to Giovanni Bellini', reprinted in
   Kelly Oliver (ed.), *The Portable Kristeva* (New York and Chichester: Columbia
   University Press, 1997), p. 301.
8. Julia Kristeva, 'Stabat Mater', in Oliver (ed.), *The Portable Kristeva*, p. 309.
9. Julia Kristeva, 'Women's Time', in Oliver (ed.), *The Portable Kristeva*, p. 364.
10. Iris Marion Young, 'Pregnant Embodiment: Subjectivity and Alienation'
    (1990), reprinted in Nancy Tuana and Rosemarie Tong (eds), *Feminism and
    Philosophy: Essential Readings in Theory, Reinterpretation and Application*
    (Boulder and Oxford: Westview Press, 1995), p. 407. Subsequent references
    are incorporated into the text.
11. Elizabeth Nihell, *A Treatise on the Art of Midwifery* (London: A. Morley,
    1760), p. 99.
12. Fay Weldon, *Puffball* (1980) (London: Coronet, 1982), p. 128. Subsequent
    references are incorporated into the text.

13. See, for example, Rosalind Petchesky, 'Foetal Images: The Power of Visual Culture in the Politics of Reproduction', in Michelle Stanworth (ed.), *Reproductive Technologies: Gender, Motherhood and Medicine* (Minneapolis: University of Minnesota Press, 1987); Susan Merrill Squier, *Babies in Bottles: Twentieth-Century Visions of Reproductive Technologies* (New Brunswick: Rutgers University Press, 1991); Laury Oaks, 'Smoke-Filled Wombs and Fragile Fetuses: The Social Politics of Fetal Representation', in *Signs: Journal of Women in Culture and Society*, 26, 1 (2000).

14. Sandra Matthews and Laura Wexler, *Pregnant Pictures* (London: Routledge, 2000), pp. 198–9.

15. *Life* (30 April 1965).

16. Imogen Tyler, 'Skin-tight: Celebrity, Pregnancy and Subjectivity', in Sara Ahmed and Jackie Stacey (eds), *Thinking Through the Skin* (London: Routledge, 2001), pp. 78–9.

17. See Marjorie Tew, *Safer Childbirth? A Critical History of Maternity Care*, second edition (London: Chapman and Hall, 1995), pp.127–30, for a discussion of this issue. It should be noted, however, that it is extremely difficult to reach a judgement about the value of screening programmes. Any calculation must balance elements which are, it could be argued, incommensurable (economic cost versus the saving of an individual life, to take the most obvious example). Antenatal care could be considered the prototype for many subsequent screening programmes (for example, screening for breast and prostate cancer), concerning the value of which there is considerable disagreement.

18. Rosalind Petchesky, 'Foetal Images: The Power of Visual Culture in the Politics of Reproduction', in Stanworth (ed.), *Reproductive Technologies*, p. 62.

19. Jane Green, *Babyville* (2001) (London: Penguin, 2002), p. 249.

20. See G.S. Dawes, F. Borruto, A. Zacutti and A. Zacutti Jr (eds), *Fetal Autonomy and Adaptation* (Chichester: John Wiley & Sons, 1990), which collects key papers in this field.

21. Alexander McCall Smith, 'Fetal Medicine: Legal and Ethical Implications', in S.L. Barron and D.F. Roberts (eds), *Issues in Fetal Medicine: Proceedings of the Twenty-Ninth Annual Symposium of the Galton Insititute, London 1992* (Basingstoke: Macmillan, in association with the Galton Institute, 1995), p. 164.

22. Rachel Cusk, *A Life's Work: On Becoming a Mother* (London: Fourth Estate, 2001), pp. 29–30. Subsequent references are incorporated into the text.

23. McCall Smith, 'Fetal Medicine', pp. 165–6. Subsequent references are incorporated into the text. The principle of 'bodily integrity' has dominated discussion of the respective rights of mother and foetus. In 'A Defence of Abortion' (*Philosophy and Public Affairs* 1, 1971, pp. 47–66), Judith Jarvis Thomson proposed that pregnancy might be considered in terms of an 'attached violinist': imagine, she suggested, that you wake up one morning and discover that you have been kidnapped and a famous violinist has been attached to your body. He is using your kidneys and will need to do so for the next nine months, otherwise he will die. Have you any obligation to preserve his life? Of course, this analogy leaves out of account the fact that pregnancy usually involves a degree of choice, but Thomson's emphasis on

the degree of physical dependence involved in gestation has been influential. See Jennifer Mather Saul, *Feminism: Issues and Arguments* (Oxford: Oxford University Press, 2003), chapter 4, for a discussion of this.

24. Clare Williams, Priscilla Alderson and Bobbie Farsides, 'Is Nondirectiveness Possible within the Context of Antenatal Screening and Testing?', *Social Science and Medicine*, 54, 3 (February 2002), p. 343.

25. M. Stacey, 'The New Genetics: A Feminist View', in T. Marteau and M. Richards (eds), *The Troubled Helix* (Cambridge: Cambridge University Press, 1996), pp. 331–49.

26. Mary Warnock, *Making Babies: Is There a Right to Have Children?* (Oxford: Oxford University Press, 2002), p. 56. Subsequent references will be incorporated into the text.

27. See the review article by R.F.A. Weber, F.H. Pierik, G.R. Dohle and A. Burdof, 'Environmental Influences on Male Reproduction', *BUJ International* 89 (2002), pp. 143–8.

28. Rachel Morris, *Ella and the Mothers* (London: Sceptre, 1997), p. 95.

29. Cathy Thomasson, the mother of this baby, gives a vivid account of his first weeks in hospital in Joanna Moorhead, *New Generations: 40 Years of Birth in Britain* (Cambridge: HMSO in collaboration with National Childbirth Trust Publishing, 1996). She writes: 'we knew there wasn't much chance we'd ever take him home, so we just took one day at a time and prayed for a miracle. He was so tiny he didn't even look like a real baby – more like a tiny monkey, covered with this dark hair. He was so early his eyes were still fused, like a kitten's – it wasn't until around 26 weeks that first one, then the other, opened and he looked at us for the first time ... It wasn't until he was eight weeks old that I got my first cuddle. It was an amazing moment – he was still covered in wires and attached to lots of machines. But it seemed a really important milestone' (p. 86).

30. Kaplan, *Motherhood and Representation*, p. 181.

31. The surrogate mother in this case, Mary Beth Whitehead, has written an account of it from her point of view. See Mary Beth Whitehead (with Loretta Schwartz-Nobel), *A Mother's Story: The Truth About the Baby M Case* (New York: St. Martin's Press, 1989).

32. Naomi Mitchison, *Solution Three* (1975), with an afterword by Susan M. Squier (New York: The Feminist Press at The City University of New York, 1995), p. 153. Subsequent references will be incorporated into the text.

33. As Squier has pointed out, Mitchison's ideas about the interaction between the cell nucleus and cytoplasm draw on the work of the embryologist C.H. Waddington, with whom she was also friendly. See Squier, *Babies in Bottles*, pp. 189–90.

34. Doris Lessing, *The Fifth Child* (1988) (London: Flamingo, 2001), p. 52. Subsequent references are incorporated into the text.

35. For example, research has been carried out into the use of animal tissue to repair damaged human heart valves.

36. Anthony Giddens, *The Transformation of Intimacy: Sexuality, Love and Eroticism in Modern Societies* (Cambridge: Polity Press, 1992), p. 27.

37. Richard Berthoud, Stephen McKay and Karen Rowlingson, 'Becoming a Single Mother', in Susan McRae (ed.), *Changing Britain: Families and Households in the 1990s* (Oxford: Oxford University Press, 1999), pp. 354–73.

This study combined quantitative and qualitative analysis, including interviews with 44 lone mothers. Subsequent references will be incorporated into the text.

38. The term 'baby hunger' comes from Sylvia Ann Hewlett's book *Babyhunger: The New Battle for Motherhood* (London: Atlantic Books, 2002). In this she argues that a large number of successful professional women are failing to have children, not because they do not want them, but because of the irreconcilable demands of a career and childbearing/rearing. When such women reach early middle age, according to Hewlett, their childlessness causes a melancholy yearning – 'baby hunger'.

39. Maeve Haran, *All That She Wants* (1998) (London: Warner Books, 1999).

40. Jane Green, *Babyville* (2001) (London: Penguin, 2002).

41. Morris, *Ella and the Mothers*, p. 111. See Whitehead, *A Mother's Story*, pp. 112–13.

42. See Robert Winston, *Getting Pregnant: The Complete Guide to Fertility and Infertility* (London: Pan Books, 1993), p. 311.

43. See Janelle S. Taylor, 'Of Sonograms and Baby Prams: Prenatal Diagnosis, Pregnancy, and Consumption', *Feminist Studies* 26, 2 (Summer 2000), p. 392. Subsequent references are incorporated into the text. Discussions of reproduction as production can be found in Emily Martin, *The Woman in the Body: A Cultural Analysis of Reproduction* (Boston: Beacon Press, 1987); Ann Oakley, *The Captured Womb: A History of the Medical Care of Pregnant Women* (Oxford: Blackwell, 1984); Barbara Katz Rothman, *Re-creating Motherhood: Ideology and Technology in a Patriarchal Society* (New York: W.W. Norton, 1989).

44. Iris Marion Young, 'Pregnant Embodiment: Subjectivity and Alienation', in Tuana and Tong, *Feminism and Philosophy*, p. 408.

45. The cover image of Demi Moore was covered by a plain wrapper when *Vanity Fair* went on sale in the US, as it was feared it would be considered indecent.

46. Sandra Matthews and Laura Wexler, *Pregnant Pictures* (London: Routledge, 2000), p. 203.

47. Celia Lury, *Consumer Culture* (Cambridge: Polity Press, 1996), p. 77.

48. See Carol Smart and Bren Neale, '"I Hadn't Really Thought About It": New Identities/New Fatherhoods', in Julie Seymour and Paul Bagguley, *Relating Intimacies: Power and Resistance* (Basingstoke: Macmillan, 1999), p. 127.

49. Quoted in Lury, *Consumer Culture*, p. 5.

50. These statistics are taken from the introduction to McRae (ed.), *Changing Britain*, p. 7.

Bibliography

Acton, William, *The Functions and Disorders of the Reproductive Organs in Childhood, Youth, Adult Age, and Advanced Life, Considered in their Physiological, Social, and Moral Relations* (London: J. and A. Churchill, 1875).

Ahmed, Sara and Jackie Stacey (eds), *Thinking Through the Skin* (London: Routledge, 2001).

Anzieu, Didier, *The Skin Ego: A Psychoanalytic Approach to the Self*, trans. Chris Turner (New Haven: Yale University Press, 1989).

Appignanesi, Lisa and John Forrester, *Freud's Women* (London: Virago, 1993).

Armstrong, Isobel, Joseph Bristow and Cath Sharrock (eds), *Nineteenth-Century Women Poets: An Oxford Anthology* (Oxford: Clarendon Press, 1996).

Austen, Jane, *Sense and Sensibility* (1811), ed. Mary Lascelles (London: Dent, 1967).

Bagnold, Enid, *The Squire* (1938) (London: Virago, 1987).

Baird, Dugald, 'The Evolution of Modern Obstetrics', *The Lancet*, Vol. 2 (July–December 1960), pp. 557–64, 609–14.

Ballantyne, J. W., 'A Plea for a Pro-Maternity Hospital', *British Medical Journal* (6 April 1901), pp. 813–14.

___ *Antenatal Pathology and Hygiene: The Embryo* (Edinburgh: William Green & Sons, 1904).

___ pamphlet reprinted from the *Journal of Obstetrics and Gynaecology of the British Empire*, 'The "Byrth of Mankynde" (Its Author and Editions)' (London and Manchester: Sherratt and Hughes, 1906).

___ *Expectant Motherhood: Its Supervision and Hygiene* (London, New York, Toronto and Melbourne: Cassell and Company, 1914).

Barker, David, *The Best Start in Life: How a Woman's Diet Can Protect her Child from Disease in Later Life* (London: Century Books, 2003).

Barker, David J. P., 'The Malnourished Baby and Infant', in *Type 2 Diabetes: The Thrifty Phenotype, British Medical Bulletin*, ed. David J. P. Barker, vol. 60 (2001), pp. 69–88.

Barrett-Browning, Elizabeth, *Aurora Leigh* (1857), ed. Cora Kaplan (London: The Women's Press, 1978).

Barron, S.L. and D.F. Roberts (eds), *Issues in Fetal Medicine: Proceedings of the Twenty-Ninth Annual Symposium of the Galton Institute, London 1992* (Basingstoke: Macmillan, in association with The Galton Institute, 1995).

Berthoud, Richard, Stephen McKay and Karen Rowlingson, 'Becoming a Single Mother', in McRae, Susan (ed.), *Changing Britain: Families and Households in the 1990s* (Oxford: Oxford University Press, 1999), pp. 354–73.

Bewell, Alan, 'An Issue of Monstrous Desire: *Frankenstein* and Obstetrics', *Yale Journal of Criticism* 2, 1 (1988).

Blackwell, Elizabeth, *The Human Element in Sex: Being a Medical Enquiry into the Relation of Sexual Physiology to Christian Morality* (London: J. and A. Churchill, 1894).

Borch-Jacobsen, Mikkel, *Remembering Anna O: A Century of Mystification*, trans. Kirby Olson in collaboration with Xavier Callahan and the author (New York and London: Routledge, 1996).

Bronfen, Elizabeth, *Over Her Dead Body: Death, Femininity and the Aesthetic* (Manchester: Manchester University Press, 1992).

Brontë, Emily, *Wuthering Heights* (1847) (Harmondsworth: Penguin, 1988).

Browne, F.J., *Antenatal and Postnatal Care* (London: J. and A. Churchill, 1935).

Brumberg, Joan Jacobs, *Fasting Girls: The Emergence of Anorexia Nervosa as a Modern Disease* (Cambridge, Mass. and London: Harvard University Press, 1988).

Buchan, William, *Domestic Medicine or, a Treatise on the Prevention and Cure of Diseases by Regimen and Simple Medicines*, second edition (London: W. Strachan, and T. Cadell; Edinburgh: A. Kincaid & W. Creech, and J. Balfour, 1772).

Bunting, Evelyn M. (ed.), *A School for Mothers* (London: Horace Marshall and Son, 1907).

Burrows, George Man, *Commentaries on the Causes, Forms, Symptoms, and Treatment, Moral and Medical, of Insanity* (London: Thomas and George Underwood, 1828).

Byatt, A.S., *The Virgin in the Garden* (1978) (Harmondsworth: Penguin, 1981).

Byatt, A.S., *Still Life* (1985) (Harmondsworth: Penguin, 1986).

Bynum, W.F. and Roy Porter (eds), *William Hunter and the Eighteenth-Century Medical World* (Cambridge: Cambridge University Press, 1985).

Campbell, Janet Campbell, *The Protection of Motherhood* (London: HMSO, 1927).

Campbell, Stuart (ed.), *Ultrasound in Obstetrics and Gynaecology: Recent Advances*, book version of *Clinics in Obstetrics and Gynaecology*, Vol. 10, No. 3 (December 1983) (London, Philadelphia and Toronto: W.B. Saunders, 1983).

Campion, Sarah, *National Baby* (London: Ernest Benn, 1950).

Carlile, Richard, *Every Woman's Book; or, What is Love?* (London: published by the author, 1828).

Carroll, David (ed.), *George Eliot: The Critical Heritage* (London: Routledge and Kegan Paul, 1971).

Carter, Angela, *Nights at the Circus* (1984) (London: Vintage, 1994).

Chapple, J.A.V. and Arthur Pollard (eds), *The Letters of Mrs Gaskell* (Manchester: Manchester University Press, 1966).

Chavasse, Henry Pye, *Advice to a Wife on the Management of her Own Health and on the Treatment of Some of the Complaints Incidental to Pregnancy, Labour, and Suckling, with an Introductory Chapter Especially Addressed to a Young Wife*, twelfth edition (London: J. and A. Churchill, 1877).

Cherry, Deborah, *Painting Women: Victorian Women Artists* (London: Routledge, 1993).

Creed, Barbara, 'Horror and the Monstrous-Feminine: An Imaginary Abjection', *Screen*, Vol. 27, No. 1 (January–February 1986), pp. 44–70.

Cusk, Rachel, *A Life's Work: On Becoming a Mother* (London: Fourth Estate, 2001).

Dakin, W.F., *A Handbook of Midwifery* (London, New York and Bombay: Longman, Green and Co., 1897).

Dale Owen, Robert, *Moral Physiology; or, a Brief and Plain Treatise on The Population Question* (1830) (London: J. Watson, 1846).

Darwin, Charles, *The Descent of Man and Selection in Relation to Sex* (1871) (New York: Hurst and Company, 1875).

Darwin, Erasmus, *Zoonomia: Or, The Laws of Organic Life*, 2 vols (London: J. Johnson, 1794).

Davidoff, Leonore and Catherine Hall, '"The Hidden Investment": Women and the Enterprise', in Pamela Sharpe (ed.), *Women's Work: The English Experience 1650–1914* (London: Arnold, 1998), pp. 239–93.

___*Family Fortunes: Men and women of the English middle class, 1780–1850* (London: Hutchinson, 1987).

Davin, Anna, 'Imperialism and Motherhood', *History Workshop*, Vol. 5 (Spring 1978), pp. 9–65.

Dawes, G.S., F. Borruto, A, Zacutti and A. Zacutti Jr (eds), *Fetal Autonomy and Adaptation* (Chichester: John Wiley & Sons, 1990).

Delavenay, Emile, *D.H. Lawrence: The Man and His Work, The Formative Years: 1885–1919* (London: Heinemann, 1972).

Denman, Thomas, *An Introduction to the Practice of Midwifery*, 2 vols (London: J. Johnson, 1788).

Deutsch, Helene, 'The Psychology of Women in Relation to the Functions of Reproduction' (1924), in R. Fliess, *The Psychoanalytic Reader* (London: Hogarth Press, 1950).

Donnison, Jean, *Midwives and Medical Men: A History of Inter-Professional Rivalries and Women's Rights* (London: Heinemann, 1977).

Douglas, Mary, *Purity and Danger: An Analysis of Concepts of Pollution and Taboo* (Harmondsworth: Pelican Books, 1970).

Egerton, George, *Keynotes and Discords* (1893) (London: Virago, 1983).

Eliot, George, *Adam Bede* (1859) (New York: Random House, 2002).

Ellmann, Maud, *The Hunger Artists: Starving, Writing and Imprisonment* (London: Virago, 1993).

Elwin, Malcolm, *The Noels and the Milbankes: Their Letters for Twenty-Five Years, 1767–1792* (London: Macdonald, 1967).

Feminist Review Collective (ed.), *Sexuality: A Reader* (London: Virago, 1987).

Firestone, Shulamith, *The Dialectic of Sex: The Case for a Feminist Revolution* (1970) (London: Jonathan Cape, 1971).

Fletcher, Loraine, *Charlotte Smith: A Critical Biography* (Basingstoke: Palgrave, 1998).

Foucault, Michel, *The Birth of the Clinic: An Archaeology of Medical Perception*, trans. A.M. Sheridan (London: Routledge, 1997).

___*The History of Sexuality: Volume One, An Introduction* (Harmondsworth: Penguin, 1990).

Fox, Douglas, *The Signs, Disorders and Management of Pregnancy: the Treatment to be Adopted During and After Confinement; and the Management and Disorders of Children. Written Expressly for the Use of Females* (Derby: Henry Mozley & Sons, 1834).

Freud, Sigmund and Joseph Breuer, Penguin Freud Library 3, *Studies on Hysteria* (Harmondsworth: Penguin, 1988).

Freud, Sigmund, Penguin Freud Library 11, *On Metapsychology* (Harmondsworth: Penguin, 1984).

Fulford, Roger (ed.), *Dearest Child: Letters between Queen Victoria and the Princess Royal, 1858–1861* (London: Evans Brothers, 1964).

Garet, Garrett, *Ouroboros, of the Mechanical Extension of Mankind* (London: Kegan Paul, Trench, Trubner & Co. Ltd, 1926).

Gaskell, Elizabeth, *Ruth* (1853) (Oxford: Oxford World's Classics, 1998).

Giddens, Anthony, *The Transformation of Intimacy: Sexuality, Love and Eroticism in Modern Societies* (Cambridge: Polity Press, 1992).

Gilbert, Sandra M. and Susan Gubar, *The Madwoman in the Attic: The Woman Writer and the Nineteenth-Century Literary Imagination*, second edition (New Haven and London: Yale University Press, 2000).

Gillis, John R., *For Better, For Worse: British Marriages 1600 to the Present* (New York and Oxford: Oxford University Press, 1985).

Gilman, Charlotte Perkins, *Herland* (1915) (London: The Women's Press, 1979).

Gilroy, Amanda, '"Candid Advice to the Fair Sex": or, the politics of maternity in late eighteenth-century Britain', in Avril Horner and Angela Keane (eds), *Body Matters: Feminism, Textuality, Corporeality* (Manchester: Manchester University Press, 2000).

Gleadle, Kathryn (ed.), *Radical Writing on Women, 1800–1850: An Anthology* (Basingstoke: Palgrave Macmillan, 2002).

Graham, Thomas John, *Modern Domestic Medicine*, second edition (London: Simpkin & Marshall, 1827).

Grand, Sarah, *The Heavenly Twins* (1893) (London: William Heinemann, 1895).

Granville, Augustus Bozzi, *A Report of the Practice of Midwifery at the Westminster General Dispensary, During 1818; including new classification of labours, abortions, female complaints, etc...*(London: Burgess and Hill, 1819).

Green, Jane, *Babyville* (2001) (London: Penguin, 2002).

Greer, Germaine, *The Female Eunuch* (1970) (London: Flamingo, 1999).

Greer, Germaine, *The Whole Woman* (1999) (London: Anchor, 2000).

Grigg, John, *Advice to the Female Sex in General, Particularly those in a State of Pregnancy and Lying-in: The Complaints incident to their respective Situations are specified, and Treatment recommended, Agreeable to Modern Practice* (Bath: S. Hazard, 1789).

Haight, Gordon, *George Eliot: A Biography* (Oxford: Clarendon Press, 1968).

Haldane, Charlotte, *Man's World* (London: Chatto and Windus, 1926).

___*Motherhood and Its Enemies* (London: Chatto and Windus, 1927).

___*Truth Will Out* (London: Weidenfeld and Nicolson, 1949).

Haldane, J.B.S., *Daedalus or Science and the Future* (London: Kegan Paul, Trench, Trubner & Co., Ltd, 1924).

Hall, Marion H., P.K. Ching and I. MacGillivray, 'Is Routine Antenatal Care Worthwhile?', *The Lancet*, Vol. 2 (July–December 1980), pp. 78–80.

Hamilton, Alexander, *A Treatise of Midwifery Comprehending the Management of Female Complaints, and the Treatment of Children in Early Infancy...Divested of Technical Terms and Abstruse Theories* (London: J. Murray; Edinburgh: Dickson, Creech and Elliot, 1781).

Hanson, Clare, 'Save the Mothers? Representations of Pregnancy in the 1930s' in *Literature and History* 12, 2 (Autumn 2003).

Haran, Maeve, *All That She Wants* (1998) (London: Warner Books, 1999).

Hays, Mary, *The Victim of Prejudice* (1799), ed. Eleanor Ty (Ontario, New York and Cardiff; Broadview Press, 1994).

Hewlett, Sylvia Ann, *Babyhunger: The New Battle for Motherhood* (London: Atlantic Books, 2002).

Holland, Eardley, R.C. Jewsbury and Wilfred Sheldon, *A Doctor to a Mother: The Management of Maternal and Infant Health* (London: Edward Arnold, 1933).

Horney, Karen, 'The Flight from Womanhood' (1926), in *Feminine Psychology* (New York: Norton, 1967).

Hunter, William, *Anatomia Uteri Humani Gravidi: Tabulis Illustrata* (Birmingham; John Baskerville, 1774).

___'On the Uncertainty of the Signs of Murder in the Case of Bastard Children' (London: J. Callow, 1812), p. 6. Paper read to the Medical Society, 14 July 1783.

Huxley, Aldous, 'A Note on Eugenics', in *Proper Studies* (London: Chatto and Windus, 1927).

Huxley, Aldous, *Brave New World* (1932), with an introduction by David Bradshaw (London: Flamingo, 1994).

Jacobus, Mary, 'Is There a Woman in This Text?', *New Literary History* 14 (1982), pp. 117–41.

Johnson, Barbara, *A World of Difference* (Baltimore and London: Johns Hopkins University Press, 1987).

Joint Committee of the Royal College of Obstetricians and Gynaecologists and the Population Investigation Committee, *Maternity in Great Britain* (Oxford: Oxford University Press, 1948).

Jones, Ernest, *The Young Freud, 1856–1900* (London: Hogarth Press, 1956).

Kaplan, E. Ann, *Motherhood and Representation: The Mother in Popular Culture and Melodrama* (London: Routledge, 1992).

Keller, Evelyn Fox, *The Century of the Gene* (Cambridge, Mass. and London: Harvard University Press, 2000).

Kitzinger, Sheila, *The Experience of Childbirth*, revised edition (Harmondsworth: Penguin, 1967).

Kristeva, Julia, 'Motherhood According to Giovanni Bellini', reprinted in Kelly Oliver (ed.), *The Portable Kristeva* (New York and Chichester: Columbia University Press, 1997), pp. 301–7.

___'Stabat Mater', reprinted in Oliver (ed.), *The Portable Kristeva*, pp. 308–31.

___'Women's Time', reprinted in Oliver (ed.), *The Portable Kristeva*, pp. 349–69.

Lacan, Jacques 'The Mirror Stage as Formative of the Function of the I as Revealed in Psychoanalytic Experience', in *Ecrits: A Selection*, trans. Alan Sheridan (London: Tavistock, 1977).

Laënnec, E.T.H., *Treatise on Mediate Auscultation and Diseases of the Lung and Heart*, trans. J. Forbes, second edition (1827).

Laqueur, Thomas, 'Bodies, Details, and the Humanitarian Narrative', in Lynn Hunt (ed.), *The New Cultural History* (Berkeley and London: University of California Press, 1989), pp. 176–204.

Lawrence, C.J., 'William Buchan: Medicine Laid Open', *Medical History* Vol. 19 (1975), pp. 20–35.

___ *Medicine in the Making of Modern Britain 1700–1920* (London: Routledge, 1994).

Lawrence, D.H., *The Rainbow* (1915) (Harmondsworth: Penguin, 1972).

Laycock, Thomas, *Mind and Brain: or, The Correlations of Consciousness and Organisation: Systematically Investigated and Applied to Philosophy, Mental Science and Practice* (London: Simpkin, Marshall and Co., 1869).

Lee, Robert, *Three Hundred Consultations in Midwifery* (London: John Churchill and Sons, 1864).

Lemione-Luccioni, Eugénie, *The Dividing of Women or Woman's Lot (Partage des Femmes)*, trans. Marie-Laure Davenport and Marie-Christine Reguis (London: Free Association Books, 1987).

Lessing, Doris, *A Proper Marriage* (1964) (St Albans: Panther Books, 1966).

___*The Fifth Child* (1988) (London: Flamingo, 2001).

___*Under My Skin: Volume One of My Autobiography, To 1949* (1994) (London: Flamingo, 1995).

Lewis, Jane, *The Politics of Motherhood* (London: Croom Helm, 1980).

Lewis, Judith Schneid, *In the Family Way: Childbearing in the British Aristocracy, 1760–1860* (New Brunswick: Rutgers University Press, 1986).

Lewis, Sarah, *Woman's Mission* (London: J.W. Parker, 1839).

Leybourne-White, Grace and Kenneth White, *Children for Britain* (London: Pilot Press, 1945).

Life (30 April 1965).

Llewelyn Davies, Margaret (ed.), *Maternity: Letters from Working Women* (1915) (London: Virago, 1978).

Loudon, Irvine, *Death in Childbirth: An International Study of Maternal Care and Maternal Mortality 1800–1950* (Oxford: Clarendon Press, 1992).

___ (ed.), *Western Medicine: An Illustrated History* (Oxford: Oxford University Press, 1997).

Lury, Celia, *Consumer Culture* (Cambridge: Polity Press, 1996).

Macfie, Ronald C., *Metanthropos, or the Future of the Body* (London: Kegan Paul, Trench, Trubner & Co. Ltd., 1928).

Malthus, Thomas, *An Essay on the Principle of Population as It Affects the Future Improvement of Society, With Remarks on the Speculations of Mr Godwin, M. Condorcet, And Other Writers* (London: J. Johnson, 1798).

Mansfield, Katherine, *In a German Pension* (1911) (Harmondsworth: Penguin, 1975).

___ *Selected Stories* (Oxford: Oxford World's Classics, 1981).

Marland, Hilary (ed.) *The Art of Midwifery: Early Modern Midwives in Europe* (London: Routledge, 1993).

Marteau, T. and M. Richards (eds), *The Troubled Helix* (Cambridge; Cambridge University Press, 1996), pp. 331–49.

Martin, Emily, *The Woman in the Body: A Cultural Analysis of Reproduction* (Boston: Beacon Press, 1987).

Martin, Emma, *The Bible No Revelation, or the Inadequacy of Language to Convey a Message from God to Man*, second edition (London: published by the author, c.1850).

Matthews, Sandra and Laura Wexler, *Pregnant Pictures* (London: Routledge, 2000).

Matus, Jill L., *Unstable Bodies: Victorian Representations of Sexuality and Maternity* (Manchester and New York: Manchester University Press, 1995).

Maudsley, Henry, *The Physiology and Pathology of Mind*, second edition (London: Macmillan and Co., 1868).

Mazumdar, Pauline, *Eugenics, Human Genetics and Human Failings* (London: Routledge, 1992).

McCall Smith, Alexander, 'Fetal Medicine: Legal and Ethical Implications', in S.L. Barron and D.F. Roberts (eds), *Issues in Fetal Medicine: Proceedings of the Twenty-Ninth Annual Symposium of the Galton Insititute, London 1992* (Basingstoke: Macmillan, in association with the Galton Institute, 1995), pp. 163–71.

McCleary, G.F., *Race Suicide?* (London: George Allen and Unwin, 1945).

McLaren, Angus, *Reproductive Rituals* (London and New York: Methuen, 1984).

McRae, Susan (ed.), *Changing Britain: Families and Households in the 1990s* (Oxford: Oxford University Press, 1999).

Mears, Martha, *The Midwife's Candid Advice to the Fair Sex: or the Pupil of Nature* (1797), A New Edition (London: Crosby and Co. and R. Faulder, 1805).

Mitchell, Juliet, *Mad Men and Medusas: Reclaiming Hysteria and the Effects of Sibling Relations on the Human Condition* (Harmondsworth: Penguin, 2000).

Mitchell, S. Weir, *Wear and Tear, or Hints for the Overworked*, fifth edition (Philadelphia: J.B. Lippincott Company, 1887).

Mitchison, Naomi, *Solution Three* (1975), with an afterword by Susan M. Squier (New York: The Feminist Press at The City University of New York, 1995).

Moers, Ellen, *Literary Women* (New York: Doubleday, 1977).

Montgomery, W.F., *An Exposition of the Signs and Symptoms of Pregnancy, the Period of Human Gestation, and the Signs of Delivery* (London: Sherwood, Gilbert, & Piper, 1837).

Moorhead, Joanna, *New Generations: 40 Years of Birth in Britain* (Cambridge: HMSO in collaboration with National Childbirth Trust Publishing Ltd., 1996).

Morris, Norman, 'Human Relations in Obstetric Practice', *The Lancet*, Vol. 1 (January–June 1960), pp. 913–15.

Morris, Rachel, *Ella and the Mothers* (London: Sceptre, 1997).

Moscucci, O., *The Science of Woman: Gynaecology and Gender in England, 1800–1929* (Cambridge: Cambridge University Press, 1990).

Murray, Janet Horowitz (ed.), *Strong- Minded Women* (Harmondsworth: Penguin, 1984).

News of the World (8 April 1928).

Nihell, Elizabeth, *A treatise on the art of midwifery. Setting forth various abuses therein, especially as to the practice with instruments: the whole serving to put all rational inquirers in a fair way of very safely forming their own judgment upon the question; what it is best to employ, in cases of pregnancy and lying-in, a man-midwife or, a midwife* (London, A. Morley, 1760).

Nordau, Max, *Degeneration*, trans. from the second edition of the German (London: William Heinemann, 1895).

Oakley, Ann, *The Captured Womb: A History of the Medical Care of Pregnant Women* (Oxford: Blackwell, 1984).

Oaks, Laury, 'Smoke-Filled Wombs and Fragile Fetuses: The Social Politics of Fetal Representation', in *Signs: Journal of Women in Culture and Society*, 26, 1 (2000), pp. 63–107.

Oliver, Kelly (ed.), *The Portable Kristeva* (New York and Chichester: Columbia University Press, 1997).

Opie, Amelia, *Adeline Mowbray* (1805) (Oxford: Oxford World's Classics, 1999).

Otis, Laura (ed.), *Literature and Science in the Nineteenth Century* (Oxford: Oxford World's Classics, 2002).

Pankhurst, Sylvia, *Save the Mothers* (London: Knopf, 1930).

Peel, Robert A. (ed.) *Essays in the History of Eugenics* (London: The Galton Institute, 1998).

Perkin, Joan, *Victorian Women* (London: John Murray, 1993).

Petchesky, Rosalind, 'Foetal Images: The Power of Visual Culture in the Politics of Reproduction', in Michelle Stanworth (ed.), *Reproductive Technologies: Gender, Motherhood and Medicine* (Minneapolis: University of Minnesota Press, 1987), pp. 57–80.

Playfair, W.S., *A Treatise on the Science and Practice of Midwifery*, third edition (London: Smith, Elder, & Co., 1880).

Porter, Roy, *The Greatest Benefit to Mankind: A Medical History of Humanity from Antiquity to the Present* (London: Fontana Press, 1999).

Power, John, *Essays on the Female Economy* (London: Burgess and Hill, 1821).

Priestley, W.O. and Horatio R. Storer (eds) *The Obstetric Memoirs and Contributions of James Y. Simpson, Professor of Midwifery in the University of Edinburgh* (Edinburgh: Adam and Charles Black, 1854).

Pritchard, James Cowles, *A Treatise on Insanity and Other Disorders Affecting the Mind* (London: Sherwood, Gilbert, and Piper, 1835).

Queen Charlotte's Practice of Obstetrics, first edition, ed. J. Bright Banister et al. (London: J. and A. Churchill, 1927).

Queen Charlotte's Textbook of Obstetrics, eighth edition, ed. G.F. Gibberd et al. (London: J. and A. Churchill, 1952).

Radcliffe Richards, Janet, *The Sceptical Feminist: A Philosophical Enquiry* (1980) (Harmondsworth: Penguin, 1988).

Read, Grantly Dick, *Natural Childbirth* (London: William Heinemann, 1933).

___ *Revelation of Childbirth* (London: Heinemann, 1942), published in the US in 1944 as *Childbirth Without Fear*. This was the title subsequently adopted in Britain.

Reid, D. and M.E. Cohen, 'Trends in Obstetrics', *Journal of the American Medical Association*, Vol. 142 (1950), pp. 615–23.

Rich, Adrienne, *Of Woman Born: Motherhood as Experience and Institution* (1976) (London: Virago, 1986).

Romero, Patricia, E. *Sylvia Pankhurst: Portrait of a Radical* (New Haven and London: Yale University Press, 1987).

Rothman, Barbara Katz, *Re-creating Motherhood: Ideology and Technology in a Patriarchal Society* (New York: W.W. Norton, 1989).

Royal Commission on Population, *Report* (London: HMSO, 1949).

Russo, Mary, *The Female Grotesque: Risk, Excess and Modernity* (London: Routledge, 1994).

Ryan, William B., *Infanticide: Its Law, Prevalence, Prevention and History* (London: J. and A. Churchill, 1862).

Saleeby, Caleb Williams, *Woman and Womanhood: A Search for Principles* (London: William Heinemann, 1912).

Saul, Jennifer Mather, *Feminism: Issues and Arguments* (Oxford: Oxford University Press, 2003).

Sebba, Anne, *Enid Bagnold: The Authorized Biography* (London: Weidenfeld and Nicolson, 1986).

Seymour, Julie and Paul Bagguley (eds), *Relating Intimacies: Power and Resistance* (Basingstoke: Macmillan, 1999).

Shelley, Mary, *Frankenstein: or The Modern Prometheus* (1818), ed. Maurice Hindle (Harmondsworth: Penguin, 1992).

Sheridan, Frances, *Memoirs of Miss Sidney Bidulph* (1761) (Oxford: Oxford World's Classics, 1999).

Shoemaker, Robert B., *Gender in English Society 1650–1850: The Emergence of Separate Spheres?* (Harlow: Longman, 1998).

Showalter, Elaine, *The Female Malady: Women, Madness and English Culture, 1830–1980* (London: Virago, 1987).

Shuttleworth, Sally, *Charlotte Brontë and Victorian Psychology* (Cambridge: Cambridge University Press, 1996).

Smart, Carol and Bren Neale, '"I Hadn't Really Thought About It": New Identities/New Fatherhoods', in Julie Seymour and Paul Bagguley, *Relating Intimacies: Power and Resistance* (Basingstoke: Macmillan, 1999), pp. 118–41.

Smellie, William, *A Treatise on the Theory and Practice of Midwifery*, 3 vols (London: D. Wilson, 1752–64).

___ *Anatomical Tables with Explanations and an Abridgement of the Practice of Midwifery, with a view to illustrate A Treatise on that Subject and Collection of Cases* (1754), A New Edition, Carefully Corrected and Revised, with Notes and Illustrations Adapted to the present Improved Method of Practise By A. Hamilton (Edinburgh: William Creech, 1787).

Smith, Adam, *An Inquiry into the Nature and Causes of the Wealth of Nations*, 2 vols, ed. R.H. Campbell, A.S. Skinner and W.B. Todd (Oxford: Clarendon Press, 1976).

Smith, Charlotte, *Montalbert: A Novel*, 3 vols (London: E. Booker, 1795).

___ *The Young Philosopher: A Novel*, in four volumes (London: T. Cadeli, Jun. and W. Davies, 1798).

Smith, R.D. (ed.), *The Writings of Anna Wickham, Free Woman and Poet* (London: Virago, 1984).

Southcott, Joanna, *Memoirs of the Life and Mission of Joanna Southcott, interspersed with Authentic Anecdotes and elucidated by Interesting Documents including the Progress of her Pregnancy detailed by herself together with the Opinions of Drs Reece and Sims to which is added a Sketch of the Rev. W. Tozer, M.J.S. embellished with a Striking Likeness of the Prophetress* (London: M. Jones, 1814).

Spencer, Herbert, *The Study of Sociology*, seventeenth edition (London: Kegan Paul, Trench, Trubner & Co., Ltd., 1894).

Spring Rice, Margery, *Working-class Wives: Their Health and Conditions*, with an Introduction by Dame Janet Campbell (Harmondsworth: Penguin, 1939).

Squier, Susan Merrill, *Babies in Bottles: Twentieth-Century Visions of Reproductive Technology* (New Brunswick, New Jersey: Rutgers University Press, 1994).

Stacey, M., 'The New Genetics: A Feminist View', in T. Marteau and M. Richards (eds), *The Troubled Helix* (Cambridge: Cambridge University Press, 1996), pp. 331–49.

Stopes, Marie, *Wise Parenthood* (1918), twelfth edition (London: G.P. Putnam's Sons, 1926).

Summers, Leigh, *Bound to Please: A History of the Victorian Corset* (Oxford: Berg, 2001).

Taylor, Barbara, *Eve and the New Jerusalem* (London: Virago, 1983).

___ *Mary Wollstonecraft and the Feminist Imagination* (Cambridge: Cambridge University Press, 2003).

Taylor, Janelle S., 'Of Sonograms and Baby Prams: Prenatal Diagnosis, Pregnancy, and Consumption', *Feminist Studies* 26, 2 (Summer 2000), pp. 391–418.

Tew, Marjorie, *Safer Childbirth? A Critical History of Maternity Care*, second edition (London: Chapman and Hall, 1995).

Theriot, Nancy, 'Diagnosing Unnatural Motherhood: Nineteenth-century Physicians and "Puerperal Insanity"', in Philip K. Wilson (ed.), *Childbirth: Changing Ideas and Practices*, Vol. 5 (New York: Garland, 1996), pp. 133–52.

Thomson, J., 'A Defence of Abortion', *Philosophy and Public Affairs* 1, 1971, pp. 47–66.

Todd, Janet (ed.), Mary Wollstonecraft, *Mary* and *Maria*; Mary Shelley, *Matilda* (Harmondsworth: Penguin, 1991).

Tuana, Nancy and Rosemarie Tong (eds), *Feminism and Philosophy: Essential Readings in Theory, Reinterpretation and Application* (Boulder and Oxford: Westview Press, 1995).

Tuke, J.B., 'On the Statistics of Puerperal Insanity as observed in the Royal Edinburgh Asylum, Morningside', *Edinburgh Medical Journal*, Vol. X (July 1864–June 1865) (Edinburgh: Oliver and Boyd, 1865), pp. 1013–28.

Tyler Smith, W., *A Manual of Obstetrics: Theoretical and Practical* (London: John Churchill, 1858).

Tyler, Imogen, 'Skin-tight: Celebrity, Pregnancy and Subjectivity', in Sara Ahmed and Jackie Stacey (eds), *Thinking Through the Skin* (London: Routledge, 2001), pp. 69–83.

Walker, Alexander, *Woman, Physiologically Considered as to Mind, Morals, Marriage, Matrimonial Slavery, Infidelity and Divorce* (London: A.H. Baily & Co., 1840).

Wardle, Ralph M. (ed.), *Collected Letters of Mary Wollstonecraft* (Ithaca, NY and London: Cornell University Press, 1979).

Warnock, Mary, *Making Babies: Is There a Right to Have Children?* (Oxford: Oxford University Press, 2002).

Weber, R.F.A., F.H. Pierik, G.R. Dohle and A. Burdof, 'Environmental Influences on Male Reproduction, ' *BUJ International* 89 (2002), pp. 143–8.

Weismann, August, *Essays Upon Heredity and Kindred Biological Problems*, 2 vols (Oxford: Clarendon Press, 1889–92).

Weldon, Fay, *Puffball* (1980) (London: Coronet, 1982).

Whitehead, Mary Beth (with Loretta Schwartz-Nobel), *A Mother's Story: The Truth About the Baby M Case* (New York: St. Martin's Press, 1989).

Williams, Clare, Priscilla Alderson and Bobbie Farsides, 'Is Nondirectiveness Possible within the Context of Antenatal Screening and Testing?', *Social Science and Medicine*, 54, 3 (February 2002), pp. 339–47.

Wilson, Adrian, *The Making of Man-Midwifery: Childbirth in England 1660–1770* (London: UCL Press, 1995).

Wilson, Philip K. (ed.), *Childbirth: Changing Ideas and Practices in Britain and America 1600 to the Present*, 5 vols (New York and London: Garland, 1996).

___'"Out of Sight, Out of Mind?": The Daniel Turner-James Blondel Dispute over the Power of the Maternal Imagination', in Wilson (ed.), *Childbirth: Changing Ideas and Practices*, Vol. 3, pp. 361–83.

Winston, Robert, *Getting Pregnant: The Complete Guide to Fertility and Infertility* (London: Pan Books, 1993).

Wollstonecraft, Mary, *Political Writings* (Oxford: Oxford World's Classics, 1994).

Wood, Ellen, *East Lynne* (1861), ed. Andrew Maunder (Peterborough, Ontario: Broadview Literary Texts, 2000).

Wyndham, John, *The Midwich Cuckoos* (1957) (Harmondsworth: Penguin, 1960).

Young, Iris Marion, 'Pregnant Embodiment: Subjectivity and Alienation', reprinted in Nancy Tuana and Rosemarie Tong (eds), *Feminism and Philosophy: Essential Readings in Theory, Reinterpretation and Application* (Boulder and Oxford: Westview Press, 1995), pp. 407–19.

Zytaruk, George J. and James T. Boulton (eds), *The Letters of D.H. Lawrence, Vol. 11, 1913–15* (Cambridge: Cambridge University Press, 1981).

Index